My Sh*t Therapist

& other mental health stories

—

Michelle Thomas

LAGOM
BOOKS FOR A BETTER BALANCED LIFE

Published by Lagom
An imprint of Bonnier Books UK
3.08, The Plaza,
535 Kings Road,
Chelsea Harbour,
London, SW10 0SZ

www.bonnierbooks.co.uk

Hardback 9781788701907
eBook 9781788701914

A CIP catalogue of this book is available from the British Library.

Designed by Envydesign Ltd
Printed and bound in Great Britain by Clays Ltd, Elcograf S.p.A.

1 3 5 7 9 10 8 6 4 2

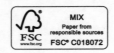

For Mam and Dad, with love and gratitude

Contents

Preface

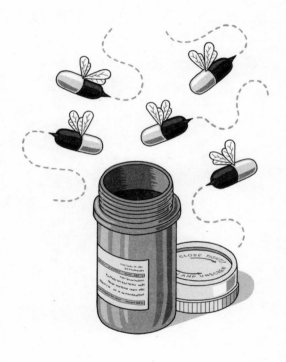

W HAT'S THE DIFFERENCE BETWEEN A NATURAL, NORMAL response to trauma and pathological mental illness?

If you're hoping that this book will answer a question that's foxed experts for decades, then you, my friend, are very much out of luck.

First of all, no one ever lies down during therapy. There's never anything to lie down on. It's always a chair, most often an Ikea special. There's always a table with a prominently placed box of off-brand tissues (you don't go for Kleenex when you get through five boxes a week). Clocks are cunningly placed so that you can't see them from your seat, but the therapist can from theirs. 'This is *your* time.' You'll hear that a lot.

One day six years ago, I started crying and couldn't stop. I crawled into bed and stayed there for nearly two weeks. It was six months before I could return to full-time work.

My name's Michelle Thomas. I'm a writer (which means that I've spent most of my career working in pubs and cafes). I'm addicted to manicures, my signature look is 'gender-fluid Sideshow Bob', and I take 20mg of citalopram, a type of antidepressant known as a selective serotonin reuptake inhibitor (SSRI), daily for anxiety and depression. I'd never planned to write a book about my mental illness. But then, I never planned to be mentally ill.

The depression I have experienced isn't just feeling low or fed up. It's the first thought to form on waking up, it's dread at leaving the oblivion of an 18-hour sleep. It's crying because you're thirsty but you can't summon the will to walk to the kitchen, take a glass, turn on the tap, fill the glass with water, turn off the tap, then drink. It's the absence of any feeling, any drive. It's collapsing onto bed, shutting the door on your parents,

3

your loved ones, the people who want to help you, because you're exhausted from carrying the weight of your own worthlessness.

Having depression doesn't mean I'm always depressed, in the same way that being allergic to bee stings doesn't mean a person is in constant anaphylactic shock. It's only when they get stung that it's a problem.

Like a person who is prone to depression, a person with a bee sting allergy can get stung at any time. Their allergy is not dependent on their life circumstances. They could win the lottery, have the body of a South Korean athlete and attend weekly murder mystery nights with Ruth Jones and Charlotte Church, and they'd *still* be allergic to bee stings. Their allergy isn't negated by terrible world events or the fact that there are many people worse off than them (and it's profoundly unhelpful to suggest that it is). Being allergic to bee stings doesn't make you a bad friend, bad parent or bad employee. It isn't indulgent or selfish: it's a chemical anomaly. If an allergic person is stung by a bee, it's important they don't feel afraid or ashamed to get help. Treatments that may relieve the effects of a bee sting for a person who is not allergic to them, such as vinegar or spit on a dock leaf, are not effective to a person who *is* allergic to bee stings. Those allergic people need an EpiPen, and in some cases professional medical attention. You can't snap out of an allergy, and a positive mental attitude, though helpful, is not an antidote.

A person who is allergic to bee stings may encounter a bee and not get stung. For example, if a friend or colleague with the allergy fears they are at risk, they might say to you, 'Hi, I'm allergic to bee stings, and there's a bee in my office. I'm going to close the window to prevent more bees coming in. I would also like to remove this enormous bouquet of flowers from my desk.' Then you could say, 'Sure thing, I'll put the bouquet in my office instead.' If that person hasn't been stung for a while, that doesn't mean they're no longer allergic. Though they may take every precaution, no one is guaranteed lifelong bee sting evasion. However, no one should live in fear of their body's response to a chemical imbalance. By encouraging people to talk openly about their allergies, and educating others about what to do if they encounter someone having an allergic reaction, we can make our gardens safer for everyone, and we can all enjoy some time in the sun.

When I was ill, I'd wake up every night between 3:30am and 5:30am. I had two options. I could lie in bed imagining – *living out* – all the terrible things that could happen to the people I love. Or I could get out of bed and write. So that's what I did. That's not what this book is. I know that would be neat, but most of what I wrote during those lonely hours was gibberish. But it gave me something to do, somewhere to put my madness, a way to contain it. To make sense of it.

The popular narrative about mental health is one of breakdown and recovery – 'I wanted to kill myself, but now I run ultra-marathons!' While every experience is valid and I applaud anyone who finds a way through their darkest moments, most people live their lives somewhere in the middle of those two binary states. They're not in crisis, but they're not coping well either. These are the moderately mad – the one in ten British adults who are prescribed antidepressants for various forms of mental illness. Some are experiencing a response to trauma or formidable stress – a bereavement, a break-up, seemingly insurmountable debt. Some have been diagnosed with more complex pathological disorders. Some, like myself, don't have a Scooby Doo what's caused their depression, but know that medication keeps them from bursting into tears at unexpected noises, or when a 'soldiers-reunited-with-their-dogs' video pops up on their Instagram feed.

So I don't know whether common mental health issues are a pathological illness or a normal human response to constantly changing life circumstances. I've tried to educate myself – I read James Davies' brilliant book *Cracked*, and was appalled to discover that some women have been prescribed Prozac to treat PMS, and that the American Psychiatric Association's *Diagnostic and Statistical Manual of Mental Disorders* now includes caffeine withdrawal and internet addiction in its canon of mental illnesses.

I spent a lot of time worrying about pathologising my own illness. Then I realised, it doesn't really matter. (I mean, in the macro sense, of course it matters. I know that Big Pharma makes billions of pounds a year from the notion that the drugs – and *only* the drugs – work.)

I take my meds because they work for me, and I feel wonky without them.

I accept that I have been ill.

But has the name I give my own madness ever helped me get out of bed?

No.

Has the nature vs nurture argument ever talked me down from having a panic attack?

No.

Maybe most of us don't need to worry about what particular label to put on the squatter in our brains. We only need to worry about how to evict it, or at least to live without fear of it burning the fucking house down.

* * *

A couple of years ago, I was a guest on a popular radio show. I was working in a cafe at the time, and a blog I'd written about being body-shamed by a Tinder date had gone viral (more on this later). This was one of a flurry of invitations I'd received to talk about my experience.

I'd just finished a quiet shift. I made myself a flat white, took off my tabard and took a seat just before the producer rang to finalise the details – what time they'd call, what kind of questions I'd be asked, what the presenter's name was (always good to know).

'There's something else I wanted to tell you, actually,' I heard her say, and then she trailed off.

'What's that?' I asked.

'I, err… actually I suffer from depression too.'

'Oh,' I said dumbly.

'Yes. I take medication for it.'

'Oh,' I said again, even dumbly-er.

'I've never told anyone. No one in my family knows. I don't think they'd understand.'

We chatted about our shared experience of mental illness for a few minutes. When and how it started. What the symptoms were. How we both tried (and failed) to beat it into submission with busy-ness. And for a long time, I just listened and gave her space to speak, and be heard. I think this is the most valuable thing I could offer and I was – and am – genuinely honoured to have been given her trust and able to help her in a small way.

This radio producer needed not only to voice her pain, but to be heard by someone who understood it. Who understood her. She didn't feel her friends, family and colleagues could offer her that (although I wonder how many of them were hiding the same secret), so she reached out to a stranger.

'I'm 54 years old and I've never told anyone, apart from my GP,' she said. 'I had to come and sit in my car to ring you because I didn't want anyone I work with to overhear. It's difficult, so thank you. What you're doing is hard, and you're helping people.'

I held the phone away for a moment so that she wouldn't hear me choke up.

'Thank you for letting me know,' I said, 'and please take care.'

We both signed off, and a few minutes later I got a cheery email confirming the details of the radio spot.

* * *

Imagine having a debilitating illness.

Imagine keeping it secret from your family, friends and colleagues.

Imagine having to hide in your car to finally tell someone you hope will understand you – a total stranger – for fear that someone you work with might find out about your mental illness.

If it were diabetes, or a sprained ankle, or a chest infection, that would be absurd. Why should a mental health issue be any more shameful?

According to the World Health Organisation, more than 300 million people worldwide are now living with depression, an increase of more than 18 per cent between 2005 and 2015. Approximately one in four people in the UK experience a mental health problem each year. The shame and stigma accompanying this makes it difficult for people to ask for help when they need it most. That's if they even recognise that they need it.

If we all sought to prioritise our mental health needs every day, the result would be far-reaching positive improvement at work, in our relationships and in wider society. I've called this book *My Sh*t Therapist* because getting an appointment to see a therapist was the first step (or mis-step) that I took in taking charge of my mental health.

I want to share what it's like to navigate life with mental illness, not just in the pole-to-pole journey from illness to wellness, but the day-to-day admin in between. Madmin, as it were. What it's like to live with a misbehaving brain. Poor mental health affects every aspect of your life, from who you choose to date and what career you think you can cope with, to what you'll have for dinner when you can't face a crowded supermarket and lack the cognitive stamina (or can't afford) to order a takeaway. I hope that this book will offer comfort and reassurance. I've included some practical strategies that have helped me recover, and still help me manage my depression when it comes to dating, working, spending and more.

This book is about my experience, which I recognise is limited. As a straight white woman, my mental illness isn't exacerbated by prejudice against my race or sexuality. I don't know what it's like to be diagnosed with schizophrenia, or psychosis, or borderline personality disorder. I'm not an addict. My depression doesn't make me violent. I can, if I choose to, hide my mental illness while others don't have that privilege. So while I'm going to be honest about my mental health story, I'll also be sharing stories that all sorts of different people have contributed. People whose mental health changed after having a baby. People who have physical illnesses that directly contribute to their mental illness. People whose mental health has changed in their 30s, 40s, 50s and beyond. People whose jobs put their physical and mental health at risk.

These people wrote to me to share their experiences, in their own words. As such, some of these stories use language that you may consider to be outdated, or ableist. 'Nuthouse'. 'Crazies'. 'Batshit'. This is the language that many of us use to discuss, process, and take ownership of our experiences.

I wanted to share their stories as accurately as possible, and while some entries have been edited for length and clarity, I've stayed as faithful as I can to their own words.

* * *

When I was very ill during a major depressive episode, I read and watched and listened to everything about depression I could get my hands on in an effort to fix myself. *God*, it was boring. This was before I discovered Matt Haig, Ruby Wax, Maggy van Eijk and a wealth of other engaging, honest, brilliant mental health writers. Most of the information I had to hand was painfully earnest, bone-dry, bland and forgettable. Frankly, it was depressing, which was the last thing I needed. While of course it's important that the topic is treated with sensitivity and respect, I wanted what I was reading to mimic the frank and honest and – dare I say? – *funny* conversations I've had with my friends about our shit brains.

Writing *My Sh*t Therapist*, hearing stories from people from every corner of the mental health spectrum, has taught me that while we can seek help from a million sources, we each have to find one that's right for us, for our particular brand of madness. I hope you find the one that's right for you.

I started writing this book because I couldn't find anything like it when I needed it most. I hope it will act as a support network and friend to those who may be in the loneliest and most frightening period of their lives. For loved ones who need help to understand. For people like that frightened radio producer. I hope it will help you talk about mental illness with your family, friends, colleagues and partners. I hope it will help to change the way we think and talk about our minds.

And if you're reading this between 3:30am and 5:30am, this book is especially for you.

1

My Shit Diagnosis

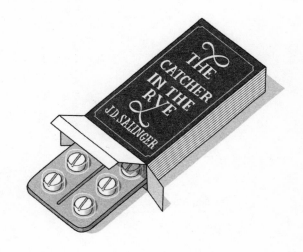

YEARS BEFORE I SAW A THERAPIST FOR MY MENTAL ILLNESS, I was prescribed American literature.

When I was growing up, my primary school report said, 'Michelle is eight, going on 40.' Even at that tender age, I felt old-headed and ill at ease with my classmates. By the age of 15 I felt like an alien – at school, in my town, in the confines of my own skin. My home town is a small, rural place in Snowdonia, North Wales. Its beauty attracts thousands of visitors per year, but very few of them stay, and very few residents leave. I was lonely and depressed. I didn't know that at the time, of course. Everything I experienced – the isolation, the horrible, corrosive anxiety, my profound hatred of my body that meant I stayed home from school two days a week to avoid PE – I put down to my inherent, weird *wrongness*. Like many teenagers, I was also deeply solipsistic. I truly believed that no one else could possibly begin to understand, let alone empathise. I lived in terror of losing the few friends I had, so I couldn't tell anyone how I really felt and I assumed that I was the only person who'd ever felt this way.

One night after school, the children's BBC show *Blue Peter* was on. We weren't a *Blue Peter* household, but I half-listened as the presenter chirruped that today's episode was a special about autism. I'd never heard the word before, so I tuned in with curiosity. What Katy Hill did next stopped my heart.

She said, 'Autistic people are very intelligent, but they find it hard to make friends.'

In the Welsh language, the word for 'relate' – *perthyn* – also means 'belong'. Katy's words related to my situation, but they also *belonged* to me. They resonated with every dark and lonely part of me. My experience had a name.

I was autistic.

I could have wept with relief.

I hurried upstairs, scrawled the word 'AUTISM' on a scrap of paper and hid it in my jewellery box. I looked up the condition in the British Medical Association's *Family Health Encyclopedia* and as I read the description of autism, I felt it fill my brain and smooth over every chip and crack in my fragmented identity. There I was. There really *was* something different about me. Now I had the proof. [1]

I booked an appointment with our GP without my parents knowing – a high-risk strategy in a small town. The doctor I saw had no doubt seen countless teenage girls without their parents' knowledge.

'What can I do for you?' he asked kindly.

I looked him straight in the eye and confidently announced, 'I think I have autism.'

I understand now that the clarity and directness of this announcement isn't typically associated with the condition, and that it may have been evidence that I was not, in fact, autistic. But I didn't know that at the time.

The doctor was very quiet for a very long time, but when he spoke there was the same even-keeled note in his voice.

'I see,' he said. 'And why do you think that?'

My confidence faltered. Then the tears came. And I told him everything. How I felt clever and stupid at the same time. How hard I found it to relate to people my own age. How hard it was to make friends, to connect with people. How lonely and anxious and sad and *tired* I felt all the time – all day, every day.

---

1 Please note, dear reader, that this says a lot more about my view of my 15-year-old self than it did or does about my view of autistic people.

He nodded sagely, and listened to every single word, and didn't speak until I'd finished.

Just as I began to sense the first creeping shadow of shame at the edges of my misery, he spoke again, and his words gently shooed those feelings away. 'Have you ever read the novel *The Catcher in the Rye?*'

I'd never heard of it. I shook my head.

He took a scrap of paper from his notebook – not dissimilar to the one I'd scrawled my misdiagnosis on – and purposefully wrote JD SALINGER, *THE CATCHER IN THE RYE*, then handed it to me like a prescription.

'Read this. It'll make you feel normal.'

There are some who might think it unwise to prescribe American literature for teenage depression. And in fairness, they're not wrong. But in my case, neither was Dr B. He'd known me since before I was born, and he gave me exactly the treatment I needed. He didn't laugh at me. He didn't tell me off for wasting his time. He didn't put me on antidepressants (although I would take medication years later, I didn't need them then). And most importantly, he did not tell my parents. He somehow understood that what I needed was to be shown a way of life outside that of my stifling small town.

It didn't work, of course. It's a great novel, but as a 15-year-old girl in rural Wales I found it hard to relate to a 15-year-old boy in New York who steals credit cards and hires a sex worker. Where would I even find a sex worker? The nearest big town was Wrexham, and that was a two-hour bus journey away. I worked a Saturday job in a cafe for something like £1.50 an hour. How much would a sex worker cost? The Salinger solution prompted more questions than it answered.

It can be reductive and condescending to prescribe a book as a cure for mental illness. But Dr B knew that for me and millions before and after me, books are the gateway to a million ideas and experiences that have to be imagined before they are realised. And for that I will be eternally, hopelessly grateful to him, because at the time, his advice was enough.

And sometimes, it's enough now. It's enough to feel Ray Davies or David Bowie or Marian Keyes or Nick Cave or Roxane Gay reach through the screen or the page or the airwaves or the canvas and take my hand and say *I know. I know. But it's going to be all right*.

But more on the life-affirming power of art and music and books and films shortly.

What *The Exorcist* taught me about anxiety

Anxiety isn't the same as feeling nervous before a job interview. It's scanning every room you walk into for potential threats. It's knowing that you'll fail that exam, despite your achieving consistently high marks. It's being close to tears all day because you were ten minutes late for work and you're wracked with guilt and self-loathing. It's finding a tiny blemish on your breast and lying awake, weeping silently so as not to wake your partner, convinced that you have cancer, and playing the moment when you have to tell your family over and over in your mind. It's second- and third- and fourth-guessing every single decision you make every single day.

The score for the film *The Exorcist* is laced with layers of low-volume, low-frequency noise that provokes fear in our primal brains. Swarms of angry bees. Disturbing industrial sounds. So, throughout the movie, not just in the shockingly visceral scenes that made the film infamous, the audience is triggered into a fear response even when there's no visible threat.

This is my experience of anxiety: a perception of an invisible threat that I can't explain because I'm not conscious of the cause. And because I'm perceiving a threat, my brain invents scenarios where that fear could be put to good use.

* * *

A few years ago, I was in the grip of a horrible depressive episode. I'd been in my bedroom all day, and now it was 5:30pm – too late to do anything, but too early to go back to bed and sleep for another 100 years. *Exercise*, I thought, vaguely. *That'll tire me out, then I can go back to bed.* So, I bundled myself up and paced the streets of South London. It was dark and cold. My breath felt shallow and frantic, and I tried to force it into the rhythm of my feet as I walked – two steps in, four steps out.

In the rush-hour traffic I saw a cyclist. My brain conjured a vivid image of him being knocked off his bike. In real life, he cycled on, but in my mind's eye he was now under a car, bleeding to death and crying for his mother.

I flinched, burrowed my mouth and nose into my scarf and marched on.

In real life, a priest walked by. Now she was incorporated into this grim fantasy, giving the boy his last rites as his blood soaked into her robe.

Huh, I thought, *I AM mad.*

I kept walking and let the lurid imaginings play themselves out. I turned right down a tree-lined street, away from the cars and the cyclists and the people. Two steps in, four steps out.

* * *

I asked my online community what happened the first time they sought help to deal with their mental health.

Harald
If I jump now, everything will be easier

My mental illness evolved over many years – high-energy periods of success followed by deep, dark days of depression, lack of self-worth and doubt. It got worse year after year.

One day I was looking from the kitchen window in our apartment block, five floors above the backyard, and thought, *If I jump now, everything will be easier.* I was so shocked when I realised what I had just thought that the very next day I made an appointment with a doctor.

Anonymous
So what if she's depressed? She's running, isn't she!?

The first GP I saw asked me why I had been having troubles with my mental health. I told him about my abusive relationship, about the difficulty I had finding motivation in life, my loneliness, my helplessness. He listened as if he'd come in right at the end of a radio programme and was trying to catch the ending, but wasn't really that interested. When I mentioned that I went running, he jumped into action: 'Have you joined a local running group? I find they are most helpful with giving one a sense of community at times like this.'

He then asked if I'd tried reading some self-help books. I had, incidentally, when going through CBT [cognitive behavioural therapy] a few years earlier. I told him I found them condescending and unhelpful, to which he replied, 'There are studies that suggest otherwise.'

Because I told him I wasn't self-harming anymore and, because I told him I went running, he didn't seem to be fussed about asking me anything else. So what if she's depressed? She's running, isn't she!? She must be OK. He asked me what I did when I got thoughts about self-harming, and I told him I went for a cigarette, which was, when you thought about it, just another form of self-harm. He laughed at this and said, 'Probably a better one, though.'

I left that consultation feeling disaffected, deflated, angry and even more helpless, so I'm phoning a local charity to see if they can help me. I might pay for private counselling although I can't afford it. It sucks to be depressed.

Pete

I started to feel like my whole life was like
The Truman Show

From manic depression to sheer batshit crazies, my family have had a good dose of it all over the years. One uncle once said it is great fun going into the 'nuthouse' and he thought everyone should try it at some time. He'd been institutionalised two or three times himself.

My first inkling that something wasn't quite right occurred

when I was sat down watching TV. I started to think the TV show was about me. I started to feel like my whole life was some fecked-up TV episode, like *The Truman Show*. I promptly went to the doctor's and was diagnosed with stress and depression.

Alice

Today, for the first time, I have asked for help

I went to the doctor today for the first time about my mental health. I think I have been living with depression for 18 years (since I was at uni). It has lingered in the background, whispering to me. I didn't know why I felt so at war with myself all the time, and the term 'depression' didn't seem to fit. I had good things in my life, I liked being around people, and I could usually find things to laugh about. I just thought I needed to be better at looking after myself, appreciating what I had and be more resilient.

When the dark thoughts come, I wish to cease to exist. I wish to be the one to get cancer. I am so angry at myself for this. I feel like I'm living life through smoked glass and not in carefree technicolour.

I also believed that my circumstances determine my happiness. I have chased and chased change and new things in the hope it would fix me. The problem of Me. But it hasn't, and I realise that it won't. Because depression has lied to me. It has told me it's my fault, it has told me I'm alone and it has deceived me into thinking it doesn't exist.

But today, for the first time, I have asked for help. Even if I feel like a fraud for claiming to be unwell, this is the best way to take care of myself. I have no idea what medication will do to me, but I am tired of pushing for change externally. I intend to smash that smoked glass, in the hope I'll find something on the other side.

J
Because I'm quite a laughy, smiley person on the outside, people struggle to understand

My GP was actually my rugby coach as well. I felt like shit and was constantly thinking about death. I never seriously attempted suicide, but I thought about it loads. I'd take medication, but I'd look up the maximum amount you could take before you'd die, and I'd take that. It was just really odd. So I went to see my rugby coach. It took a few times because every time I went, he'd say, 'You're not depressed, I've seen you play.' He kept telling me there was nothing wrong with me, and I'd have to argue and say, 'I think there is.' Because I'm quite a laughy, smiley person on the outside, people struggle to understand and take me seriously when I say I'm depressed.

Gregg
I knew I had to get help when I didn't have the energy to look after myself

It's a creeping long-term thing. Everything was super-super-hard. When I was really ill, I stopped doing things I enjoy, like writing and making music. I knew there was something up, because those things usually make me happy and get me excited, but I couldn't get excited about anything. My way of viewing things was so off-kilter that everything was boring. Not even that – boredom is like waiting for a bus for ten minutes with nothing to do. This was like the widest net of existential despair. Nothing I could ever think of or do in the future would be interesting, there was no point to anything. I was smoking too much weed, because I had nothing to do and it passed the time. Not good. I knew I had to get help [from a mental health professional] when I didn't have the energy to shower and look after myself.

2

My Shit Decade

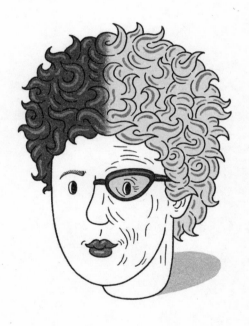

I GRADUATED IN 2009, JUST AS THE RECESSION WAS PEAKING. I moved to Bristol, and started several odd jobs. Initially there were four – cafe in the morning, office gruntery in the afternoon, theatre tech (lights on, lights off, nothing too… well, technical), and performing on alternate nights. Yep, I was an actor in an original, immersive theatre production. A *leading* actor, I'll have you know. It was actually quite good – the theatre critic Lyn Gardner called my performance 'genuinely thrilling' in the *Guardian*. I loved the show, and I was very proud to land my first professional role, but after two months of working 14-hour days – mind-killing menial work and insanely intensive rehearsals where I was often given little more direction than, 'Michelle, your lover has abandoned his pregnant wife and is on his way for a knee-trembler with you. It's wet fanny time, yeah?' – and despite my best efforts, barely covering my rent in my illegal sublet, I was exhausted.

I've never kept a regular diary, but I've written sporadically since I was a kid as a way of processing my thoughts. A kind of Depression Diary, if you will. There's an instant relief that comes from shifting any concerns or worries from my brain onto the page. During this stressful period, my feverish scribbles documented a slide into despair, as overwork and financial insecurity began to take their toll, with seven-day working weeks stacked one of top of the next and opening nights looming.

Here's an extract:

This will pass and everything will fall into place
I feel anxious about the show, and inadequate about my
performance

My Sh*t Therapist

I'm horribly dependent on and grateful for praise
I'm nauseous, light-headed and constantly on the verge of tears
My moods change so rapidly, even as I write this I'm not sure
    what's true
I need a holiday
I need to gain some perspective
This is my body, my chemicals and hormones sending all the
    wrong messages
This can be fixed
My chest is tight all the time
I need to relax
This will pass
I need to not feel guilty for doing nothing
I need to not worry
I need to look after myself
I need to remember that dark thoughts are like clouds
    and will eventually roll past
I need to take a few days off next week
I need to remember that I am in control and that this
    can be managed
I need to remember that I do this because I enjoy it
I need to remember that my sister loves me and is coming
    to see my show and is bringing her boyfriend
I need to remember my parents love me
I need to remember that I look lovely when I make a
    bit of effort
I need to not drink for a while
I need to take a big fuck-it pill
Enjoy yourself
Ring someone who knows how this feels

I have been constantly working/rehearsing for two months
I've run myself into the ground
I need to remember my achievements
I need to remember that no one is judging me
I need to remember that I have overcome this before
I need to see my breaking point and listen to myself.

One night I finally cracked and phoned home in tears. My mum wasn't home, so, in a never-before-encountered twist, it was my dad who bore the brunt of my messy meltdown, as I sobbed about how unhappy I was, how my life wasn't taking shape the way I knew it was meant to, and how scared I was that I'd never achieve all the things I wanted to, even though I wasn't entirely sure what those things were.

My dad – a stoic, still-waters-run-deep Welshman – was having none of it.

'Now, listen. Listen to your dad,' he commanded.

I hushed up immediately. I knew he was about to say something spectacular because he'd addressed himself in the third person.

'When I was your age,' he began wistfully, 'all I wanted to do was drive coaches all over Europe, but I didn't get my HGV licence. No matter how many times I tried, I kept failing the test. Instead, I drove an ambulance for years. Now, your dad's retired. He's got himself a little part-time job driving coaches, and he's over the moon! He's been to Poland, Holland, Germany! He's driven a double-decker around the Arc de Triomphe! The point is, you don't get everything you want when you want it, *cariad*. It takes time. But you'll get there, like your dad did.'

My dad saved lives for the best part of 30 years. I can't imagine the things he's seen, with no opportunity to decompress or process any of it. Now at 60-odd, he was getting paid to go on holiday and get treated like a bit of eye candy (urgh, gross) by the white-haired ladies on Women's Institute coach trips to Amsterdam and Krakow.

My dad had reminded me that it takes time to realise who you want to be, and more time to take steps to become that person. Not everyone has a true north – a vocation, a thing that they know they must work towards doing every day forever. Although I admire true-north people – Lauren Laverne was in a band at 16, Caitlin Moran wrote her first novel at the same age – some of us take the scenic route. Sarah Millican did her first stand-up gig at 29. Viola Davis's film breakthrough came when she was 43. Vera Wang designed her first dress at 40. No one outside the scientific community had heard of Charles Darwin until he published *On the Origin of Species* aged 50, and Julia Child produced her groundbreaking first cookbook when she was 49. The fact is that some things in life take a long time to happen, and maybe they feel sweeter when we have the emotional maturity to truly appreciate them. I certainly think so. If I'd escaped rural Wales for London at 18 to try and kick-start a career in the theatre, I'd almost certainly have got myself into some staggeringly ill-advised and unseemly scrapes. But then, maybe there's a downside that I'm not seeing...

Last year, on the first day of a family-oriented festival, I was lounging on the grass near a group of kids in their early teens.

'Oh God,' I heard one of them sigh, 'I feel like I'm missing out on so much, just sitting here. I'm just not making the most of it.'

It was around 11:00am, and while there were various book recitals and poetry readings going on, this was a *child*, who felt guilty for taking half an hour to sit idle on a blazing summer's day. That attitude, that fear of missing out (FOMO) is too often borne through our teens and well into our 20s. Now I'm in my 30s, I can't see a bright young thing without wanting to grip them by the shoulders and bellow, wild-eyed: 'ENJOY THESE YEARS, WITH YOUR ACHE-FREE JOINTS AND EYES THAT DON'T LOOK LIKE YOU'VE STUBBED CIGARETTES OUT ON THEM IF YOU GET LESS THAN EIGHT HOURS' SLEEP.' We're bombarded with messages by the media that idealise youth while telling us that the only valid experience of young adulthood must involve BOOZE and SHAGGING and FUN FUN FUN all the time. You must also have a bottomless fund for the right make-up and the right clothes and the gallons and gallons of grog. This relentless worship of youth amounts to horrific pressure to make every single moment special. The social assumption is that we will be paired up with our One True Soulmate by the age of 30 and hurry to spawn. The other is that once you settle down and have babies, your time for exploring and learning is over (if I see one more list of 'Things to do before you turn 30', windpipes *will* be crushed). So, in the 12 years between 18 and 30, you MUST:

* Travel the world.
* Choose an area of it that you want to live in for the rest of your life.

* Learn everything you want to learn (unless you want to be a – shudder – *mature student*).
* Land your dream job.
* Find The One who you'll happily stick with until you're dead.

All this while nursing the hangover from the perpetual partying, which you'll also have to find time to document on social media, so that all the other 18–30s know that you're on course.

But if you end up spending four years at uni, then another two in an OK job that cover bills, beer and new boots, but is not the life-enhancing career you dream of, that's half of your youth already gone. No wonder we say youth is wasted on the young. They're too paralysed with fear to enjoy it.

At 21, it's easy to believe the lie that if you don't have your dream job by 25, or are at least working towards it, you've failed. With the cost of living seeming to balloon every week, it's getting more and more difficult to leave home and get a job – ANY job – and make ends meet, never mind set up your own business or make money from creative endeavours. Not many can afford to work for free for 'experience', or worse, 'exposure'.

When there's so much pressure to do it all and to do it *now*, it's hard to keep the things that matter in perspective – health, happiness, balance, family, relationships, above all, spending time doing things that make you feel good. The days are long, but the years are short. If you spend your youth aiming to do things you love and that are important to you – baking, writing, gigging, competitive spear-fishing, whatever – you'll be happier. And that, I think, is the true measure of success.

Top ten things that make me happy

1. Getting my nails done. There's no satisfaction like flawless nails. There's no joy like admiring your fingers as you go about your chores; doing laundry (ooh, clickety-clack!), filling the dishwasher (ooh, they look so nice against the white plates!), emptying the bins (hello again, shiny ovals of joy!). When I feel low, the first thing I abandon is personal presentation. I stop caring what I wear or what my hair looks like. Applying make-up is a chore, an expulsion of energy that could be better spent hating myself. But whatever I'm doing, whether I'm out on the pull or pulling pints, when my nails look beautiful, I feel nice. My manicures are proof that I care enough about my own happiness to spend time and money on it. They are one of the everyday ways I keep my joy-muscles limber, and I've got a freshly painted middle finger for anyone who says that's flippant or unworthy.

2. Emails 'from' my three-year-old niece. My mum sends them. She doesn't know how to attach more than one image at a time, so every few weeks my inbox is flooded with 50 emails, each with one picture and a little note.

   'Hello, Aunty Michelle. Can't wait to come and see you xxxx.'
   'Would you like to share my ice cream?'
   'Wearing my cha-cha heels to watch *Strictly*.'

3. Seeing my friends do well. One of the ugliest tropes about female friendships is the idea that we should feel threatened or jealous when our friends become successful. I get a genuine buzz out of seeing people I like doing what they really love, because I know how hard they've worked to get there.

4. Getting lifts from my dad in his car. We sit in silence. Sometimes he'll whistle, quietly. It's lush.

5. New bedding, new pyjamas, new socks, things that *feel* nice. If I were an eccentric billionaire playgirl, I'd never wear the same pair of socks twice.

6. My home. It's tiny. There's no freezer, no bath, no outside space and no washing machine, and it's so freakishly affordable that I live in fear that my landlord will cop on and start charging me twice the rent, but for now it's *mine*. I'm too old, too weird, and too grumpy for house-shares (more on this later). Being able to close the door on the world and revel in sweet, sweet solitude, finding a tiny corner of a busy city that I can call my own without bankrupting myself, is pure bliss.

7. Graveyards. Is it too late to become a goth in your 30s? I missed my chance as a teen. I find them very peaceful. My top three? Well, since you ask: Highgate in London, Arnos Vale in Bristol, and a teeny, tiny one that's being slowly eroded in

Heysham, Lancashire, as if the sea is claiming back its dead. Say what you will about the Victorians, but they built a damn good cemetery.

8. Public libraries. All the books you can eat, for free. And one of the only indoor spaces open to the public where you're not obliged to spend any money. When work dried up in Bristol, I moved in with my boyfriend in Preston. I was on the dole for three months before I finally bagged a part-time job in a local cafe. Being unemployed meant that my self-esteem was so low it was practically subterranean, but borrowing and returning books gave me a reason to leave the flat when I was alone and the bed crooned lasciviously at me to crawl back into its cottony embrace. To this day, nothing calms me like a half-day in my local library with a few books and a notepad. Which brings me to…

9. Writing by hand. I can't draw, and I don't have a curator's eye that knows how to make colours and shapes and textures look beautiful, but I do have nice handwriting. As I've said, I mostly write as a way of processing and documenting my thoughts. The act of converting the fog behind your eyes into marks on paper is immensely clarifying. It doesn't have to make sense. It doesn't have to be spell-checked. No one ever has to read it – not even you. I like to write in A4 sketchbooks with a spiral top, and I prefer coloured pens that help separate and

compartmentalise my thoughts. If you take away nothing else from this book, please – get yourself to Paperchase or Waterstones or your fave local indie shop, get yourself a *nice* notebook and a pen that feels *right*, and empty your soul into it. I guarantee that your heart will be lighter and your mind will be calmer when you've finished.

10. Going to a natural history museum and checking out the names of the animals and birds. Zorilla. Bosman's potto. Civet. Major Mitchell's cockatoo. Ocellated turkey. Paradoxical frog. Resplendent quetzal. Grizzled skipper. Great jacamar. Beautiful nuthatch. Some long-dead biologist who was charged with cataloguing 50 types of birds, fish and small mammals gave them glorious, flamboyant, grandiose titles instead of perfunctory, forgettable monikers, and that never fails to cheer me up.

It's worth mentioning that the first time I tried to write this list, I failed. I was Sad, and I couldn't think of anything that made me Not Sad, because I couldn't imagine *being* Not Sad. But when the sadness lifted, I was able to identify the habits and the relationships and the *gifts* that I could give myself, for very little cost and effort, that make me feel good. Writing this list felt like stockpiling weapons in case my emotional balance is overthrown by a depression-led coup. It's part of a strategy for wellness – a flawed and scrappy one, yes, but it's a hard-won start.

So take your nice pen and your nice notebook, and make your own list. And put it somewhere you'll be able to find it when you desperately need to be reminded of the things that make you feel better. Photograph it, scrapbook it, share the shit out of it. The items won't cure a mental illness, but they might alleviate the symptoms, and sometimes that's enough.

The main reason youth is idolised in our culture is its undeniable beauty. Gorgeous thick hair, as yet untainted by a decade (or two, or three) of bleach and heat. Glowing, plump post-adolescent skin. Bright eyes, wet noses, waggy tails. The cruellest thing about getting older is not that our bodies change, but that we see how cute we used to be, and remember how much we hated ourselves even then.

Of course, we have regrets – that haircut, those tragic eyebrows, the low-slung jeans with a G-string peeking out 'alluringly'. My biggest regret is a £160 pair of Kurt Geiger thigh-high stiletto boots. JLo wore them to the Video Music Awards, I wore them to a *very* classy Wrexham establishment called Liquid & Envy. The heels were toothpick-thin, the zip barely closed over my chubby chicken-drummer calves, and they clung to my legs like sausage skins. I wore them with denim skirts, mismatched summer dresses, and on one unfortunate occasion, I wore them to a christening (I'd like to take this moment to apologise to my sister for that one). I desperately wanted to be a Sexy Woman, and they were Sexy Woman boots. I thought if I wore them I'd absorb their sexiness through osmosis, but all they did was amplify my blundering girlhood.

I don't know a single thirty-something who would go back and live their 20s again without the perspective that comes with ageing. They're simply too fraught with anxiety, insecurity and too much cheap booze. My depression kicked in properly in my late 20s, but in hindsight I can see its foreshadowing long before then.

I was 21 when I started at uni, three years older than many of my peers, so I felt I had some catching up to do. I forced myself to be a social butterfly, to be an extrovert. All my life, at school, at college, then in horrible relationships, I had made myself smaller, quieter, turning down the volume on my intellect, my curiosity and my sexuality, and now I was unrestricted. I snogged *loads* of boys. It wasn't Sodom and Gomorrah – it was Preston, Lancashire – but at the time it felt like a bit of a breakthrough. For the first time I was Having Fun, the way young people are supposed to Have Fun. And since I had the self-control of Amy Winehouse on her birthday week and the metabolism of a hummingbird (OK, that's one thing I *do* miss about my 20s), the party never stopped. Hungover? Get drunk! Sad? Get drunk! Happy? Get drunk! Uncertain how to navigate young adult friendships because you struggled to make friends through your childhood and teens? Chug-chug-chug!

Unsurprisingly, the friendships that formed around these hazy, rosé-and-lager-fuelled sessions didn't stand the test of time. And in my third year, when I mistakenly kissed the wrong boy on a night out, all the threads that connected me to the women I'd formed my first adult friendships with fell away like cobwebs.

Being dumped by a lover is awful. Being dumped by a friend is hideous. Being cast out by an entire friendship group is… intolerable.

Lectures were tense. After a few icy exchanges I stopped going out altogether (and honestly, by that point it probably did me a world of good to have the excuse not to hurt myself with more booze). My grades increased dramatically (funny, that). Thank Odin I wasn't on Facebook at the time. I can't imagine how painful dealing with the fallout online would have been.

A year after the event, a couple of girls from the group reached out to me, but it was too late to resuscitate those friendships. After the hurt had gone, I was left with sadness and no small amount of anger.

Sometimes I'm still sad that there are very few people in my life from that period. Very occasionally I'll stalk them on social. One of them is pregnant now. She looks happy and in love. And I'm sincerely happy for her.

But if we reconnected, we'd have to resurrect that old conflict. That's hard enough when you're feeling chipper, but when you're nursing a broken heart and your anxiety is in overdrive, it's almost impossible. Sometimes, for the sake of your sanity, it's best to simply cut the past loose, and move on.

* * *

We know that our bodies and physical health change over the course of our lifetime. I wanted to know how others' mental health has changed throughout their life.

Kiah

You can feel lost in your own body, which is a totally strange place to be

My life has been privileged since birth. I've wanted for nothing and live a life full of support and love. I have been lucky enough to study and work in multiple countries, from Europe to the Middle East, and I travel for the pleasure of exploring new places. I have no sad story to tell or any trauma in my life to blame for my poor mental health. The only conclusion I can come to is that the 20s are the most fucked-up and confusing time of anyone's life. You have to reinvent yourself and conform to society's idea of what an adult should be.

By the time I was 21, I was living in Dubai with a great job and every opportunity at my feet, but I was shadowed by a big ugly depressive fog that lingers over me to this day (though the 50mg of sertraline [an antidepressant] helps).

Not knowing what you want can be turmoil enough if you place too much focus on it. It can cause a void, an empty place; you don't know who you really are and what your life means, because you have changed so rapidly in such a short space of time that your mind can't keep up anymore.

Sometimes there is no trauma, and it's OK for there to be no reason for your depression. It doesn't matter that you are only 20 or 21 and have no reason to feel the way you do. You are entitled to feel your emotions whether they are positive or negative, and the people that tell you to 'Get a grip, you have a great life' – well, just tell them to fuck off. You can feel lost in your own body, which is a totally strange place to be. Four years on from my first depressive episode, I'm still on the road to recovery and have fought hard to get here. Recovery doesn't just happen with some magic pills; it takes a lot of soul-searching, therapy, writing, reading, crying, talking and travelling to find what you are looking for. But the answer is always inside you, and only when you get to that place can recovery truly start.

Harald

*When I confided in my best friend about my depression,
he called it a mid-life crisis. I didn't mention it again*

When I was between 30 and 40 I'd had some therapy, but nothing really worked out. Shortly before I reached 40, I started thinking about suicide and started to take medication. When I confided in my best friend about my depression, he called it a mid-life crisis. I didn't mention it again. Between the ages of 40 and 45 I suffered two major depressive episodes, which contributed to the end of my marriage of 25 years. Since then I've struggled to find the right partner, but at 55 I finally think I am getting to the core of the problem and am optimistic that I might have some happy years left.

Nicholas

*I wasn't forced to fully confront my depression
until I tried to kill myself*

At 15, I was obsessed with death. Serial killers, Gothic literature, the conspiracy theories surrounding Kurt Cobain's death. I ground my teeth, had constant headaches and insomnia, felt lethargic and was very angry about American foreign policy. But I was also fully in love with the romanticism of being sad. It was a flag I could wrap myself in; I could glory in my magical melancholy.

Because I had first been diagnosed as suffering from depression during my teens, it meant that in my mid-20s I clocked up my depression to youthful indulgence, claiming for years that I was not clinically depressed nor had any kind of mental illness. I would say 'I'm just sad,' which was correct, but it was not a diagnosis.

I wasn't forced to fully confront my depression until I tried to kill myself.

Zoe
I had buried myself

In my mid-20s I moved 200 miles from my home town to go to uni. Over three years my tutors implied that I had an undesirable temperament. I was defensive, the way I dressed was too masculine, I didn't compliment people enough. I was advised to be more like people on my course.

Before this, I reckon I had been pretty confident, happy in my opinions, my lifestyle, my thing. Now, suddenly, I started trying to be someone I wasn't, because I had been told that that person wasn't so great. I started to withdraw, to hide myself behind a more 'desirable' front. When I met people, I would model myself on them, adapt to their tastes, agree with their choices, their opinions. Soon there was hardly anything left. I didn't dare choose a film, order a drink, request a song. I ate things I didn't like, went to places I didn't want to visit, generally overrode myself in order to not stick my head above the parapet. I looked at my friends and wondered why I didn't want to do the things they did, why I was 'failing at life'. I had buried myself.

I'm now in my 40s and have only recently realised what I've been doing for this whole time. I still do it; a lot of the time it's just easier, but at least now I can catch myself and make the switch. I'm also pretty pissed off that I did this to myself for the whole of my 30s.

I'm also the parent of a very strong, opinionated small child, and I hated that I was trying to subdue her spirit, stop her from being herself, and I couldn't forgive myself for that. So I'm working on it.

Jules

Dad always thought I was 'the light in the room'

One of the hardest parts of coming to terms with my mental illness, for me, was telling my parents. My mum had already noticed that I wasn't myself, but I had dismissed her observation by saying it was 'just stress'. I didn't want to disappoint them, and I didn't want them to worry more than they already did/do. But I had to be honest. I had spent too much of my life hiding my sexual orientation and quite frankly it was exhausting, I didn't want to spend years hiding my mental ill health. So I opted to tell them via social media, because I knew I wouldn't be able to get through a phone call without crying, and reassured them that I was going to be OK. Nevertheless, my parents came to visit me the next day. They claimed they were 'down South' visiting my sister. We had a very honest emotional discussion about how I was feeling. My dad wanted to know why I hadn't told them sooner; he was upset that I had felt that I couldn't, and he also found it hard to believe I was depressed, because he'd always thought I was 'the light in the room'. I told him I am still that person, and always will be. I felt so relieved that they knew and that I didn't have to pretend anymore.

Sol

I know I'm not alone

I had my son when I was 22, and no one helped me. Not my mother, my father – no one. Now, one week before his 18th birthday, he's leaving. He needs his own space. I cry all day, every day. I work in an open kitchen and customers can see me all the time, so I can't hide my tears. But he's not sad; he's grown up. I went to the doctor and said I needed help and I went back to therapy. I have another younger son and I worry I don't spend enough time with him. It's time to look after my family. Now I know I'm not alone, although sometimes it can feel like I am.

Isabel

I began to believe the only way to keep my children safe was to kill myself

At about seven months pregnant I had my first intrusive thought. I was visiting my in-laws for the weekend. I was alone in the kitchen with my nephew when I wondered, *what if I just stabbed him? What if I am possessed? What if I lose control?* I immediately went for a walk and tried to calm myself. This was the beginning of my new normal, my new battle.

The thoughts were loud and played like a broken record. I needed constant proof that I was not evil and constant reassurance that I had never committed any harm. Despite my mental health, I had another beautiful happy baby, who would become part of my nightmare. My thoughts were now revolving around my loved ones. My mind was flooded with violent images, and in each scenario I was the monster. I was convinced I was losing my mind and ultimately feared I would kill or try to hurt my children. I was convinced I was going to end up on the news, as one of those women who just snap. I began to believe the only way to keep my children safe was to kill myself. I began to google intrusive thoughts again and found the term 'Pure O', then I found two amazing women who have guided me to the proper care that I receive now. Later I was told about exposure response prevention therapy (ERP) and I finally began to get the help I so desperately needed.

3

My Shit Job

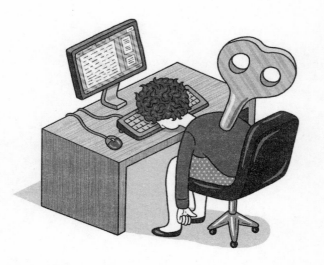

BEFORE I BECAME A WRITER/BARISTA, I WORE MANY different hats in many different jobs in theatre, comedy, opera and TV – producer, promoter, agent, stage manager, actor, runner, props mistress. These were good jobs. Fairly steady. Well-paid. The problem was that while these jobs were interesting and creative, they were only ever short-term, and none of these contracts left me any time for my *own* creative projects. I was part of some of the most prestigious venues and companies in the UK, got to travel, and met some fascinating people who were making spectacular work. But while it was my role to help others realise their own artistic endeavours, mine would naturally always take second place. Until one day I was made redundant. Living in London, I needed to line up another job, fast. I sent dozens – hundreds – of CVs a week, seemingly into the ether. I had a housemate who was unemployed at the same time. We'd stay in our rooms hunched over our laptops, grunting at each other as we crossed paths on the way to the loo or as we stood in the kitchen waiting for the kettle to boil. Apart from trawling through job websites, I had no idea what to do with myself.

This went on for a few weeks.

I needed to get out of the flat. I needed to meet and talk to others who shared my horrible predicament. I had to do something for myself, not just for the nameless, faceless judges of the sum of my character, based on two sides of A4.

It was time to take affirmative action.

It was time to consult the Big Bag for Life of Life.

My Big Bag for Life of Life

For years I'd been scribbling down ideas in notebooks and on the backs of envelopes, and putting them in a bag, to think about later. *I'll do something with all these ideas one day, when I have time,* I'd told myself. I'd lugged this growing bag of potential with me as I moved from house to house, emptying it every year or so to check its progress, then quietly refilling it. I had stacks, *reams* of the stuff.

Most of it was useless, garbage I'd accumulated over the years. Stage directions. Badly scrawled illustrations. Flyers. Tickets. Postcards. Phone numbers for costume stores, balloon makers and printers. Some terrible, *terrible* poetry.

Some of it was years and years and years old. It documented every project I'd worked on, every city I'd visited, every home I'd had, every piece of research, every shopping list, every reminder to send this or that email, every bus timetable, every piece of banal, inconsequential, irrelevant fluff that had crossed my mind to commit to paper.

On my knees, in a mire of yellowing pages, I got to work. Trawling through the pile, I salvaged what was worthwhile (photographs, bad teenage poetry), and discarded what was not (letters from a toxic ex).

I was looking for inspiration. Looking for a sign from my past self that proclaimed: This Is What You Should Do Next.

Then I found it.

Written in the corner of an old notebook from an ancient job was a single line, a barely formed thought, jotted down and immediately forgotten. It said: 'I will buy your stories for £1.'

Hmm. Buying strangers' stories for £1. Recording them,

transcribing them verbatim and sharing them online. There must be thousands of people in London who'd love to share their story – that one, special story that everyone has, about themselves or their friend or their pet or their family. It would be easy enough. And relatively cheap – for the price of an hour's yoga class I could buy stationery supplies to make a sign that read 'I will pay one pound for your story' and pay for eight stories. That would keep me occupied for a few days, and stop me from refreshing my inbox every 90 seconds to see if any job offers had miraculously dropped in my lap.

So that's what I did. My brand-new creative project – I Will Pay One Pound For Your Story – was born.

I set up a blog. I made green and gold business cards to hand out to potential participants. And on a cold day in a park in Greenwich, I collected 15 stories in two hours, recorded them on my phone, transcribed them word for word and posted them on my blog. Josh, the grumpy unemployed flatmate, came along to offer moral support. What a champ. Thanks, Josh.

The blog got some fantastic feedback. The project strengthened my CV and led to a couple of small-scale arts jobs. I repeated the experiment in other locations and posted more stories on my blog. I even planned a nationwide tour, standing around in public places in Edinburgh and West Bromwich and Southampton, listening to and paying for people's stories.

A few months later, after scraping by on these short-term contracts, I was thrilled to be offered a full-time job as an agent with a comedy company that I'd worked for as a student. It was a good job – a *dream job* – for a well-respected organisation with some big names on their books. The money wasn't great to start with, but I was assured there could be potential for a raise. And surely having a steady job in an industry I loved was better than interesting but short-term arty jobs interspersed with well-paid but crappy promo work for energy suppliers and supermarkets? It would mean postponing the tour, but I'd get around to it...

So, I was an agent now. I was initially thrilled to be part of such an exciting industry. Amazing people. Good status. Prestigious venues. Travel. Low pay. High pressure. High responsibility. Helping others' artistic goals. Long hours. No time for own creative projects.

Resentment.

Frustration.

Burnout.

Breakdown.

My mental health story

I was working with some of the biggest names in the comedy industry, hustling for gigs during the day, scouting venues during the night, getting celebs front-row seats, holding clients' hands at TV warm-up gigs and preview shows. I worked for the owner of the business, who took work calls while on holiday with his wife and kids and thought nothing of working 18-hour days, seven days a week to make his business and his name a success. He was – and is – phenomenally good at his job, and while it's easy to see why he demanded the same level of passion and commitment from his employees, it didn't seem fair of him to do so for the minimum wage. Not that I cared about my pay at first. I wanted so badly for this to be my career. I'd started off handing out flyers for this company at the Edinburgh Fringe. They'd spotted my potential, and year after year I was given more responsibility and smashed every challenge I was set with a smile. When a vacancy came up I was given the call. It seemed I'd finally found my niche.

Only I hadn't.

It was horrible.

I worked long hours, scraping for gigs in an industry over-saturated with talented people. For new clients, all of whom were based in London, I coaxed and pleaded for unpaid five-minute slots in tiny clubs in Sunderland, Plymouth and Aberystwyth. For our big hitters, I negotiated corporate shows – dinner entertainment for double-glazing specialists, insurance companies and haulage brands. These contracts paid thousands of pounds for a 15-minute set, but were always tough gigs, poorly set up in the acoustically challenged dining halls of London's finest hotels (the ones you will have heard of), in front of an uninterested and often dangerously pissed audience.

I turned up to one of these gigs with a client, a stand-up called… oh, I dunno, let's say Dave. I immediately knew it was going to be a disaster. The venue was an opulently cavernous dining hall in a big-name, five-star hotel in Paddington. The acoustics guaranteed that conversation couldn't be heard from one table to another, which is ideal if you're a filthy-rich patron regaling your companions with scandalous stories you wouldn't want to share with the room at large, but less so if it's literally your job to be heard by all 300 guests, half of whom are seated with their backs to the stage.

I tried to manage Dave's nerves backstage with soothing

words and snacks. We could hear the crowd getting more and more uproarious.

Finally it was time for Dave to do his set. He was introduced by the company director, who tried and failed to silence his employees.

Dave begins. He is a brilliant, brilliant stand-up, which is why he's being paid an obscene amount to do these gigs. But this audience doesn't want to see him. Half of them literally *can't* see him – they've been guzzling Prosecco on the company tab for the last four hours.

But he's played drunken audiences before. He opens up with a sweet gag about their industry and they start to settle down. I feel a tiny bloom of relief in my chest. Maybe it'll be all right? All he has to do is get through the next 15 minutes.

The audience ROARS in approval.

Thank *Christ*. He's got them on side, and he hasn't even delivered the punchline yet.

And then the grim reality hits me.

The suddenly much livelier crowd aren't responding to Dave. They're being served dinner.

Waiters cut across the stage in front of him, and soon the sound of clinking crockery, glasses and cutlery filled the room, along with 300 chairs being shuffled forward and drinks orders being boomed at servers. In mere minutes, the tiny bit of gravitas and attention Dave had clawed from this crowd evaporated. Now he was being resolutely ignored. He kept plugging away, but it was no use. Every second he remained on stage was agony.

Eventually – and if I'm honest, mercifully – he gave up.

'Right. I think I'm finished,' he said stoutly.

No response from the crowd.

Dave quietly plodded off the stage. No one appeared to notice, except the manager who'd booked him, and who was now glancing at me quizzically.

My heart was in my eyeballs.

I marched over to him and sternly explained that Dave had done his best in extremely difficult circumstances. 'We'll send you the invoice in full shortly,' I said curtly.

Although at first he tried to protest, he was genuinely too sozzled to give a shit.

'Fair 'nuff,' he grinned sloppily.

Now all I had to do was manage the fragile ego of a man who was fighting back tears of anger and humiliation. I was dreading the debrief with my boss. I had a horrible feeling that somehow, some way, this would end up being all my fault.

* * *

My stint in that company was the most agonising and miserable period of my life. I ate nothing but junk. I slept badly. I never relaxed, was never *able* to relax. I was desperate to do well, desperate for the you-did-good-kid hand on my shoulder. And it was killing me.

I ignored the symptoms of my depression for months. Looking back, I can recognise a pattern of upheaval, a breadcrumbs trail of cortisol-drenched anxiety that began around eight months before my nuclear fallout of a breakdown. Alongside starting this new job, the following events had occurred:

* My dad had a minor stroke (from which he fully recovered almost immediately, but it had an

immeasurable impact on our family. Dad's NEVER ill. He once dropped a breezeblock on his hand, and we had to beg him for three days to get his broken fingers looked at by a doctor).

* I moved house
* I moved in with a partner for the first time
* I worked another season at the Edinburgh Fringe Festival – a maddening, spectacular, joyous and nerve-shredding month-long whirlwind.

Each of these major, life-altering events happened weeks apart, with no recovery time in between. In less than a year, I was a wreck. I was exhausted. I cried at EVERYTHING. I made small, silly mistakes at work because my concentration was shot to pieces, but I'd berate myself for being useless. I kept saying to myself and my co-workers: 'I'll be fine. I'm just tired.' How many hidden problems does that innocuous phrase conceal? The epiphany came when I accompanied a client to the Christmas special of a BBC panel show. There was a fabulous buffet, free-flowing booze and a guest list that would make anybody sick with envy. Yet all I longed to do was slip home and eat dinner with my boyfriend. I remember checking my watch at 8:40pm. *He's cooked lasagne*, I thought miserably, as runners and technicians swooned over the mega-famous guests. *Other people would like this kind of thing, wouldn't they? They'd think it was a perk. They'd rather be partying with producers and commissioners and famous actors than curled up on the sofa, reeking of garlic and contentment.*

That was the moment when I realised I wasn't right for the job and nor was it right for me.

On the day I finally went mad, I had an appraisal during which I asked to become an employee at the comedy company rather than remain a freelancer. I was turned down. I had to 'further demonstrate commitment'. At this point I'd had to take out a credit card because my meagre wages didn't cover my travel expenses. That afternoon I secretly snuck out to a 'meeting' – an interview for a writing job in a theatre company, which finished at 2:30pm. I should have gone back to the office for the remainder of the working day, but I couldn't. I *couldn't* go back.

I remember suddenly feeling supernaturally tired, as if all the iron had drained from my blood. I took the Overground train home. I remember hoping that no one would talk to me, thinking that if another human so much as looked at me I'd shatter into a million pieces. That's the great thing about living in London: it doesn't take much effort to make yourself completely invisible. I clutched my bag and shrank into my seat, folding in on myself in my mind. By the time I arrived home, I had almost disappeared entirely.

How to have a breakdown

In this scene, the role of Michelle Thomas will be played by Charlize Theron. The role of Michelle's boyfriend will be played by Keanu Reeves. Michelle's boss will be played by Mark Strong.

INT. SMALL FLAT.

Living room – two cosy rocking chairs, sofa, bookshelf, television. MICHELLE enters. Drops bag on rocking chair. Sits on floor. Starts crying.

                                         CUT TO:

Hours later, MICHELLE'S BOYFRIEND comes home. She is still sitting on the floor in exactly the same spot, crying. He comforts her.

                                         CUT TO:

MICHELLE and MICHELLE'S BOYFRIEND sitting in their rocking chairs, watching TV and eating dinner. She's still crying.

                                         CUT TO:

INT. BATHROOM.
MICHELLE is in the bath. She's still crying, hiccups echoing wetly off the tiles.

                                         CUT TO:

INT. LIVING ROOM.
MICHELLE is sitting on the floor. Still crying. She has her phone in her hand. We see her messaging a friend.

                                         CUT TO:

INT. BEDROOM.
Later that night. MICHELLE is in bed, still crying.

                                         CUT TO:

The next day. MICHELLE has been offered the writing job with the theatre company. She's visibly tired and upset, but keeps her

voice even and normal on the phone to the
producer.

>   MICHELLE

That's wonderful, thank you so much, I'd love
to. Yes, I'm free for all those dates. Great,
I'll see you then. Thank you so much. Bye-
bye, bye-bye.

She hangs up. And bursts into tears again.

INT. SMALL FLAT.
A few days later. MICHELLE, on her bed, is
gearing herself up to make a call. There's a
notepad on her lap. She looks terrified.

>   MICHELLE

Hello, it's me.

>   BOSS
>   (warmly)

Hello, love. How are you feeling today?

>   MICHELLE

A bit shit, to be honest.

>   (Pause. She consults the notepad
>   for her next line)

I'm sorry, but I don't think I can come back.
I don't think I'm right for the job. And it's
not right for me.

> BOSS
> (long pause)

Oh.

> MICHELLE
> (tearful)

I'm sorry.

> (pause)

It feels like we're breaking up.

> BOSS
> (sadly)

You're right. It does.

> MICHELLE
> (squeaking)

Yes.

> BOSS

But it happens sometimes. You know, if it's not right, it's not right.

> MICHELLE

Yes. Thank you.

> BOSS

All right then. Take care, Michelle.

> MICHELLE

Thank you. Bye.

MICHELLE ends the call, curls up on her bed and bawls her face off.

What with all the crying, it was a very tedious period, as well as being properly fucking terrifying. I couldn't stand feeling so vulnerable. I was ashamed of it. So much of my self-worth was bound up in the fact that, four years after graduating from uni, I finally had what was considered to be a 'good' job, and the realisation that I'd backed the wrong horse was crushing. I liked having the phone numbers of people off the telly. I liked being the person those people came to when they wanted to get stuff done. I loved having my job, but, to my shame, I couldn't do it any longer.

In the following two weeks, there must have been pockets of time when I didn't cry. I know I went to the cinema once. I met up with friends twice in small, quiet cafes near my flat. But I can't remember a day when I wasn't so overwhelmed with grief that I didn't crawl into bed weeping silent, frightened tears.

Living with mental illness is like living in hell. Depression is a contrary little shit, too. Just when I needed to call on the backup reserves of positivity and stoicism that had seen me through countless adversity before, it sauntered in, squatted in my brain and crooned at me that I was unemployable, lazy, stupid, unimaginative, dull, unpopular and doomed, doomed, doomed.

I'd call my parents every day during the Bad Time. Sometimes the panic and despair would rise up in me even as I was talking to them. Spiralling, unravelling, choking terror. Every time, my dad would offer to drop everything and come and collect me and take me home. An 18-hour round trip from North Wales to London and back, which he was absolutely prepared to do, right then. Remembering his tenderness and concern breaks my heart afresh. My mum would talk me down with a gentle monologue, chattering about nothing in particular. I contributed little to the conversation beyond the odd 'Yes' or 'No'.

In those first terrible days, I was so low I couldn't summon the energy to walk to the kitchen for a glass of water. It must be hard to understand if you've never known that degree of hopelessness. What do you *mean*, you couldn't fetch yourself a glass of water? How can that be anything but laziness? But I'd spent so long ignoring my mental health that my body stepped in and said 'NO. You're not going there. You're not doing that. You're going back to bed.'

About 18 months after the episode at the comedy company, I started taking medication. Since then I've tried counselling, therapy, running, dieting and two major career changes. And while I'm better at managing my madness, I know it's still there. It probably always will be. And I'm starting to think that that's OK, as long as I know how to manage it.

After I had that breakdown, I paid my bills by making coffee and pulling pints for almost five years. While this gave me the opportunity to pursue my own creative writing, I started to believe that I wouldn't cope with anything more demanding. My experience with mental illness warped my view of my capabilities. So I didn't earn much.

Managing money when you have poor mental health can be a formidable challenge. According to British financial guru Martin Lewis, 40 per cent of people in the UK who have or have had mental health problems have severe or 'crisis debts'.

You're mentally ill because you're broke, and because you're broke you can't afford treatment, or even time from work to recover from your mental illness.

Two years after my time at the comedy company, I received a tax bill for £3,000. Rather, my actual tax bill was £800. The rest were £600 late-filing charges and a £1,600 penalty for failing to file a tax return.

I could have *vomited* with shock and confusion.

My mental health had improved after I started taking medication, but the side effects included impaired concentration, memory deficits, confusion and fatigue. This was on top of my anxiety disorder, which occasionally drove me to tears at work over whether or not I'd ordered enough regular-sized cup lids. And since I was paying tax on every payslip from my cafe job, it's no surprise that I'd forgotten to file the previous year's report.

So I called the tax office.

'It says my actual tax bill is £800,' I said, timidly.

'Are you calling to make the payment?' said a curt voice.

'No, I'm afraid I don't have it.'

'What do you mean, you don't have it?' the tax man demanded. He sounded genuinely angry, like I owed the money to him personally. 'Why don't you have it?'

Why didn't I have it?! After paying my household bills (including tax) I had a disposable income of roughly £107 per month. I was often overdrawn, so any extra income from the odd day leafleting or data collecting would go on bank charges. Yes, I'd failed to manage my finances. But I'd failed pretty consistently at every single endeavour, so that was nothing new, actually. I knew I'd need to pay taxes at some point, but my priority was keeping myself fed, warm and sheltered. I simply couldn't think as far ahead as the next tax year.

'I'm sorry,' I whispered.

'You can set up a direct debit to start making the payments, and you can appeal the penalties. But there's no guarantee they'll be dropped,' he warned.

I wrote a letter to HMRC, explaining my situation, my diagnosis, my medication and what I planned to do next. I pointed out that I'd overpaid tax in the two previous years, and that I was willing to double my monthly direct debit. I posted it, and prayed.

A few weeks later I came home from a busy shift to an official-looking letter. They'd replied. Acid rolled in my stomach as I opened the envelope with shaking fingers. Did I still owe them three grand? Had they redone their sums and worked out that I owed them even *more*? Could I go to prison if I didn't have the means to pay? What would I do?

I read the letter.

Again.

Again – four, five, six times.

It said they'd dropped all the fees and charges, and they had, in fact, overestimated the amount of tax I'd have to pay. I now owed them only £400, which I could pay off in manageable monthly instalments. No more interest would be charged.

I could have wept with relief. In fact, I think I may have done.

I finished paying it off a year later. Who knows? Next thing you know, I'll be sorting out my credit card bill.

Looking for jobs when you're depressed

Looking for a job when you're unemployed and need money is one of the grimmest situations you can find yourself in.

Writing your CV – a cold, loveless, two-page summation of your value as a human commodity – rarely produces a warm, fuzzy feeling. You spend hours agonising over which font to use. Calibri? Times New Roman? Surely not, for these are the fonts of drones. Of ANTS. Palatino might be a bit too fruity, but you can't go wrong with Bookman Old Style. Or can you? You're meticulously recalling and documenting every job you've ever had, even though you know in your heart of hearts that no one is ever going to read past the About Me section – an existential crisis in two adjectives. Who am I? Am I diligent and resourceful? Am I flexible and self-motivated? (If you describe yourself as 'well-presented' or list 'being a perfectionist' as your biggest weakness, you should probably take a long, hard look at yourself.)

A couple of years ago I cracked the code, though.

Picture the scene.

A man (of course) is reading a towering pile of CVs. He's intrigued by one in particular. Two neat sides of A4. Nice choice of font (Corbel. Edgy, but not too controversial). Suddenly, his breath catches in his throat. His eyes widen. Could it be…?

He grabs his phone and barks an order to an underling: 'Get me the MD, chop chop!'

He waits to be connected.

'Yes, sir, I'm sorry to disturb you, but this CV… it's… it's just… so. Damn. GOOD. Thomas, sir, first name Michelle. Corbel, sir – I know, great choice, but that's not all. It says that she works well – wait, there's more – she works well as an individual – and – oh GOD, wait until you hear this – AS PART OF A TEAM! HOW DID SHE KNOW THAT'S EXACTLY WHAT WE WERE LOOKING FOR? GET

HER IN! GET HER IN NOW! HONESTLY, JUST GIVE HER MY JOB. SHE DESERVES IT!'

Why can't we just say, 'Look, I'm skint, I'm desperate, this is my arse, this is my elbow, just give me some money, you dicks'?

How to talk to a loved one about their mental health

In this scene, the role of Michelle Thomas will be played by Maxine Peake. Mam will be played by Imelda Staunton. Dad will be played by the opera singer Bryn Terfel (aged up).

INT. MICHELLE'S BEDROOM.

Late morning. MICHELLE is sitting on her bed, opposite her window, mid-panic attack. Her spiralling, unravelling, choking terror is visible. She picks up the phone and calls her parents.

DAD'S VOICE

Hello?

MICHELLE

(into phone)

DAD! I'm having... a... I can't breathe.

DAD'S VOICE

All right, all right... Listen, do you want me to come and get you?

MICHELLE

(beat)

No.

DAD'S VOICE

All right.

(pause)

I'll get your mam.

(Mumbling as he hands over the phone
to Mam)

MAM'S VOICE

Hello love?

MICHELLE

MAM! I can't… get my breath.

MAM'S VOICE

OK, OK, just calm down, just caaalm down,
nice deep breaths now… (pause as she breathes
with MICHELLE) In… and out… just calm down,
love. That's it, big deep breaths. Is there
anything particular worrying you, love?

MICHELLE

I just woke up and I just felt awful and then
I got upset and I couldn't breathe—

MAM'S VOICE

OK, love, just calm down. Deep breaths.

During this speech, MICHELLE gradually – very

gradually – calms down. Occasionally she'll interject in the affirmative or negative, but she continues to hyperventilate, hiccup and cry throughout MAM's speech.

MAM'S VOICE

Deep breaths. Can you see any little birdies in your garden? I had a lovely one the other day. He was very smart with a black crown and a yellow belly and blue wings. He sat there bold as brass on the feeder, but then one of those big blackbirds scared him away – they are a nuisance. They're too heavy to feed on the fat balls themselves, but they scare the other little birds away. Spiteful. That's better, deep breaths. I bet you haven't remembered to feed yours, have you? They won't come if you don't feed them, you know! They like the fat balls.

MICHELLE

(snorts)

MAM'S VOICE

Oh yes… and I'm giving the garage doors a lick of paint – we're going to go for a lovely shade of aubergine, spruce them up a bit. Hmmm… (beat) Well, it's looking rather miserable outside. I haven't been out today, but when your dad nipped out for the paper he said it's gone cold.

My Shit Job

MICHELLE

I haven't been out yet.

MAM'S VOICE

What's this one now? He's not a robin, but
he's got an orange belly and he's got blue
wings and a black band around his eyes… Oh,
he is smart, aren't you?
MICHELLE moves from the bed to consult her
bird chart next to the window.

MICHELLE

He could be a nuthatch.

MAM'S VOICE

He's going for the fat balls now.

MICHELLE

Mam, please stop saying fat balls, they're
FEED balls.

MAM'S VOICE

Well, it says fat balls. They're balls of
fat, aren't they?

MICHELLE

If you keep saying fat balls it sounds
like you're saying FAT BALLS. Like you're
swearing.

MAM'S VOICE

Well, that's your imagination. Are you a bit
better now, love?

MICHELLE

Yeah, thank you. I just got a bit upset.

MAM'S VOICE

Are you sure there's nothing worrying you?

MICHELLE

No, no, I'm just a bit tired, I think. I haven't been sleeping very well, work's been a bit busy, I'm probably not eating very well – that probably doesn't help. That's all it is.

MAM'S VOICE

Oh, right. Did you get your nails done?

MICHELLE

Yeah.

MAM'S VOICE

What colour did you go for?

MICHELLE

Like a coral.

MAM'S VOICE

Very nice. I've gone for a – a pearlised – like a pearlised mango, if you like. Yes. OK, love.

(pause)

You're sure there's nothing else bothering you?

My Shit Job

(drops voice to a whisper)

Are you all right for money?

MICHELLE

Yes thanks, Mam. No, I'm all right, I'm just a bit tired. I'll be better after I've had a rest.

MAM'S VOICE

All right. I was thinking about you this week – your stars were good. Hang on, I'll get the paper. (pause) Listen to this: Leo…

MICHELLE

Mam, I'm a Taurus.

MAM'S VOICE

(reading)

Leo: 'You're ready to shock everyone, especially yourself, by just how much you achieve, now Mars gives you so much self-belief. A love relationship that faltered can get back to its best – if you want it to. Add tact to the advice you give.' Well, well.

MICHELLE

Mam. I'm a Taurus.

MAM'S VOICE

Are you? Oh. Well, it's all good advice. Maybe it'll rub off on you.

MICHELLE

Thanks, Mam.

MAM'S VOICE

That's all right. Now you relax now, chill out tonight, like you always say we should do… Don't be rushing around, that's enough to make anyone feel a bit under the weather. And have some tea, just some cornflakes or something to start with.

MICHELLE

Will do. Thanks Mam, love you. Bye.

MAM'S VOICE

Bye love, bye, bye.

MICHELLE hangs up. She's calmed down a little, but is still shaky, afraid and tearful.

FADE OUT.

How to talk to people when you're recovering from mental illness

After I was ill, I didn't work full-time for nearly nine months. Eventually I became a part-time barista in a local cafe, on a zero-hours contract. When I first started, I lived in fear of my former colleagues coming in to see me making sandwiches, wiping tables and emptying bins, trailing a whiff of bacon fat and bad life choices. Even though I was happier and less stressed than I had been for a long time, and my undemanding job meant that I could focus on my own creative projects, I felt like a failure. I was already avoiding Facebook notifications from my contemporaries. Their success turned my belly into a snake pit of seething envy.

After nine months of working from home as a writer, and odd lonely hours leafleting, working in a team of baristas in a busy cafe was a staggering culture shock. I was horrified to discover that my social skills had totally evaporated. It sounds ridiculous, but I genuinely struggled to judge how much or how little to say to customers. Even an innocent, 'How are you?' from a customer was a dilemma – was a polite, 'Fine, thanks, and yourself?' enough, or should I be honest and say, 'Please be gentle with me, I've worked at home in pyjama bottoms and a string vest for nine months and I've forgotten how humans work'?

At first it was humbling, I won't lie. My sense of self had always been connected to my job, to being an indispensable member of a team. My self-esteem was measured by how useful I was to other people. I craved the status of high-impact, visible roles, which – coupled with a good dollop of imposter syndrome – also made me feel anxious and depressed. If I wasn't useful, if I wasn't *special* because of my job, I didn't know who I was.

I had to relearn how it felt to go to the same place every day, and how to work with new people. I probably interacted with a couple of hundred customers every single day. For someone who couldn't leave the house not long before without bursting into tears, that's *huge*. And doing the same thing every day – making coffee, cooking industrial quantities of bacon, taking orders, handling money, cleaning up – is a skill. When you've been robbed of your confidence by a brush with mental illness, a job that allows you to learn these skills and rebuild that confidence is invaluable. Luckily I was working for two of the kindest, most relentlessly supportive women I've ever met. They gave me heaps of encouragement, and more responsibility as time went on, until I was managing my own little train station cafe. I'd write most afternoons, so I was creatively fulfilled and could pay my bills. It was flexible enough that I could work as many or as few hours as I wanted, so if I needed some quiet mental health time, I was always able to take it. And on the rare occasions when I needed to cancel a couple of shifts during a low patch, I could easily get my shifts covered and rest up without feeling pressurised to go back to work straight away. The world wouldn't end because I wasn't there to make coffee, there was always someone else who could.

I'd often serve the same people the same orders every day. Personally, I don't think there are many greater small, everyday tragedies than disappointing food. If my train's delayed for 45 minutes it's a setback, but if I pay £3 for a sub-par sandwich, my day is ruined. So I took pride in providing good food and good service to my regulars.

Every morning while I was preparing their orders, I'd ask them how they were. Over the course of a few months, I realised that I might be the only person to ask them that question. Once, the response was, 'Not great, actually. My husband's just asked me for a divorce.' An A&E doctor who came in after finishing his shift told me he'd lost a very young patient for the first time the night before. I was the first person he met afterwards and he needed to offload, so we chatted for a few minutes and I gave him a hug. Moments like this made me feel like I was playing a small but important role in my regulars' lives every day. Grandiose? Perhaps. But why wouldn't I take pride in providing a service that made every day a tiny bit more delicious? I enjoyed that job, and I was good at it. And as unlikely as it sounds, it played a valuable part in my recovery.

After a few years, my writing started getting attention. I was getting bits and pieces of journalism published and slowly building a portfolio. I developed my voice and my confidence, and began sharing my work on social media. I wrote an article about how working in a cafe gave me more time and freedom to be creative than a job in a so-called 'creative' industry had done, and somehow in the machinations of the global newspaper syndicates, it was read in Australia by a rock star called Damian Cowell. His assistant contacted me to ask if I would write a feature about his latest crowdfunded album. Damian had a gig in Melbourne in two weeks.

It would be great if I could go, I thought. *But I can't go. To Australia. I can't just take time off work, book a flight and travel to the other side of the planet in ten days, can I? I mean... can I?* The idea tickled a hard-to-reach spot in the back of my brain. Adventure called, louder than the wasps in my stomach telling me it was a terrible idea and that something was bound to go hideously wrong. But I had this strange and unfamiliar feeling that actually, all would be well. And all was well. All was wonderful, in fact. And I learned that when I listen to my instincts, not to my anxieties, good things can happen. Choose what you want to pursue. Find out what you have to do to get it. If you have to make sacrifices, make them.

When I returned to the UK, I knew I had to make some

changes in my life. It was time to move on. I'd been on an adventure and survived. Now it was time to think about what I wanted to do, how I wanted to live, and who I wanted to be. Sadly, it spelled the end of my long-term relationship, and I didn't want to stay in London anymore. I moved back to Bristol, and a year later I landed the job I'd always wanted, as a copywriter at an advertising agency.

* * *

At first I was terrified. This would be my first regular, grown-up Monday to Friday job in five years since I'd left the comedy company. Not only that, but I was worried about the effect a high-impact, potentially stressful role would have on my mental health.

Luckily I'd already published a few articles about my mental health and was able to be very open about it in my interview, and my new boss didn't bat an eyelid when I mentioned that I'd need to work around weekly therapy sessions. It's hard to speak to the people you're closest to about your mental health struggles, but I've found it much easier to speak to a co-worker. They don't know you personally, so you can pretend to be someone who's braver than you really feel.

Starting a new job is always a little awkward. Starting your first grown-up job in five years is on another level. But it was utterly exhilarating to put my creativity to work. As a freelance writer, I often felt as though I was shouting into the void, but here I was getting instant feedback – yes, no, change this bit, move that, does this work in radio? On TV? On a digital ad the size of a matchbox? There's no better feeling than being set a challenging brief and smashing it. I was around people, doing interesting, engaging work. I felt more like myself than I had in years.

A few months into the job the seasons changed, which always knocks me for six, head-wise. I started to feel *wonky* again. But this time, I knew better than to ignore it, and I felt secure enough in my environment not to have to hide it. Simply acknowledging that you're not at your best relieves the pressure of pretending that all is well. And it stops you from feeling guilty if your work is sub-standard, because you've made it known that you're struggling.

After a couple of days cowering at my desk, trying to rally myself, I finally sent my boss an email on my way to work after a therapy session:

Hi XXX,

I just wanted to flag up that I've been struggling with depression and anxiety for the last week. On Friday, it impacted my work – I made a lot of silly mistakes because my concentration was shot.

I'm looking forward to coming in to work today, and hopefully it won't affect my writing too much. I experience low patches like this two or three times a year. It's nothing I haven't met and dealt with before. I don't require any action from you, but just sending this email to you will help me regain some control over my symptoms.

I'm making an appointment with my GP to review my medication, and will keep you updated.

See you shortly,

M

And this was the response from my boss:

> *Thanks for letting us know – and I really respect you for doing so.*
>
> *Just say any time that you're struggling and need to take some time out, or just get out for some air.*
>
> *And no worries about making mistakes – again, just say if you're in need of a bit of extra support or consideration.*

Immediately I felt the burden of keeping up appearances lifting from my shoulders. It didn't cure my depression, but it did alleviate the symptoms, because I could focus solely on getting well, rather than hiding my illness.

I felt crappy for a few days, but it passed, like it always does.

Mental illness and work – our rights and entitlements

Recently, business leaders and unions asked the British government for mental health to be given the same weight as physical health in workplace legislation, so that first aiders could also deal with early signs of mental health problems.

You can take up to seven days in a row (this includes non-working days) without a sick note from a doctor.

According to the charity Mind, one in five people have phoned in sick due to stress, but over 90 per cent gave their employers a different reason for their absence, like a headache or a stomach upset. And of course, this is an option for you. You don't have to disclose your mental health status to anyone, but I do believe that the pressure of keeping it secret can exacerbate your symptoms. The Equality Act exists to protect you from discrimination in the workplace, and you have every right to request support when you need it. In fact, your employer is legally obliged to make 'reasonable adjustments' to accommodate your needs. The mental health charity Rethink Mental Illness have some fantastic resources to help you ask for what you need. For example, if your medication makes you drowsy, can you start and finish work an hour later? If your concentration is suffering, can your line manager adjust your workload until you're feeling better? Would it help if you worked longer hours for fewer days, or shorter shifts spread out over the week?

If you find commuting difficult because of a mental health issue and you live in the UK, Access to Work is a government-funded initiative that can help to meet your needs, like providing a support worker to accompany you on your journey to work, or even paying for noise-cancelling headphones to make public transport and open-plan offices more comfortable. Check the sources page at the end of the book to help you get what you need.

I'm very lucky to have finally found a job and a workplace that accommodate my mental health needs. It took some time, but it is without a doubt the single most important step I have taken in my recovery. The thing you will spend most of your time doing for up to 50 years of your life shapes your mental health, and that's more important than money, status, living in a sought-after city or an impressive job title.

According to Mind, workplace stress is one of the biggest causes of mental illness. So use your holidays. Take your lunch break every day. And don't stay in a toxic job that's making you ill.

* * *

I asked around to find out how mental health has impacted other people's careers and finances.

Olivia
I still battle frequent urges to harm myself

I'm a 30-year-old accountant with self-harm scars on my arm and wrist. I still battle frequent urges to harm myself, but this feels so much more taboo to talk about than other symptoms, even than suicide. Because of the crazily long NHS waiting lists for counselling, last year I was advised by my very supportive and well-meaning employers to ring the company's Employee Assistance Programme. Ten minutes into my first telephone counselling session, the therapist declared that I didn't have depression after all – I had a vitamin B12 deficiency!

I don't. I even had a blood test to check.

I love that the conversation around mental health is going strong, but I worry that it's still in its infancy and is quite sanitised. By that, I mean it's OK to have depression and anxiety, but other conditions such as schizophrenia or borderline personality disorder are rarely discussed.

Ceren
I thought I could save humanity, like a messiah

I have been hospitalised 'by force' five times. Each time, I was sacked from my job. Each time, I had to deal with the depression that comes right after mania and lasts for maybe a year.

I had my first manic episode at 22. I was at the highest high, full of energy and anxiety. I believed I could make it rain and take messages from songs and billboards. I thought we were all going to die, but I could save humanity, like a messiah. That's when I went to hospital.

I finally found a new job two months ago, teaching English. I had a bad year, but despite it all I'm getting better and better each day. And I did it all by myself. Unfortunately I could never find a compatible therapist. They just put me in a box labelled 'bipolar' and didn't see past that. They never tried actually reaching out to me. So I gave up and tried to overcome it on my own, which hurt me a lot, but I'm still here now.

Holly

I just couldn't control my anger and frustration

When my husband left me after ten years, I was in complete shock. I ended up being signed off work for two weeks. I started drinking a lot, like a bottle of wine, maybe more, every night for months. I started cutting myself at work, something I hadn't done for years. I just couldn't control my anger and frustration, and cutting gave me momentary clarity and a sense of calm, but I'd instantly regret it. Well, not at the beginning. I didn't care enough at the beginning to regret it.

They weren't deep cuts at first, just surface wounds, but one night I cut too deep and passed out.

The next day, a close friend patched me up and took me to the GP. I was already on 20mg of fluoxetine [an antidepressant], and that was doubled.

At this point I was guided by my work to a free employee counselling service. This helped me through some very dark moments. They then put me forward for six sessions of therapy, paid for by my employer. I'm very lucky. It helped a lot.

Anonymous
I once had a huge meltdown in front of my supervisor

I'm on 150mg of venlafaxine [an antidepressant] for my depression. I once had a really bad depression episode while at my boyfriend's. He took me to an emergency doctor, who said I didn't look depressed when I came through the door, and that I should have a lie-down and a good cry. He gave me a prescription for tablets to help me sleep, which I ripped up after the appointment. I once had a huge meltdown in front of my supervisor at work and told her I'd self-harmed and kept having bad thoughts. After this conversation and once I'd calmed down, they sent me back on to the shop floor. I understand that work is work and the ball has to keep rolling, but in that situation, I was in no state to go back. I had CBT [cognitive behavioural therapy], which really helped me. Now I'm not as anxious as I used to be, but I do have my depression days.

Gregg
Having to talk to people if you're in a customer-facing role is kind of nightmarish

Before I was diagnosed, I missed a lot of work because I was ill all the time. I couldn't get out of bed, never mind go to work.

I lost a bunch of jobs because I couldn't hold them down for very long. After I lost each one I'd have some downtime, start to feel a bit better, start another one, get worn down and eventually quit because I couldn't hack it.

Having a job gives you a sense of purpose, so if you're not working you feel like you're not really part of society. You're on a different timetable to everyone else. Everyone else is advancing and moving on and achieving things. And you're stuck in limbo.

Trying to work with heavy depression is horrible. Having to talk to people if you're in a customer-facing role is kind of nightmarish.

I was always broke, because I didn't have enough money for bills.

Now I work with SEN [special educational needs] children with anger issues. One day I might go in and there'll be a six-year-old girl pouring paint over the floor and stamping in it, chanting the C-word. Then a little boy will run in and call her a dickhead and they'll start throwing chairs at each other. I hear horrible stories about these children's home life. They're furious all the time because of what's happened to them. It's extremely challenging. There's not a lot of emotional support for staff. I'm used to being stressed, so weirdly I work very well in a stressful environment. I can just look at it and go, someone needs to do this job, someone needs to show these kids that not all adults are cruel or incompetent or dickheads. So I do it, then go home and relax.

Emma

I was a police officer at the London Riots

I did eight years in the Metropolitan Police in London. I bloody loved it for the first three years of my service – it was the best job in the world and I never imagined doing anything else. In August 2011 I was a police officer at the so-called London Riots. I was on duty for 23 hours one night. We were ambushed by a group throwing missiles at us after being lured in by a hoax call to a reported fight between six or seven people. As we got closer to where the 'fight' was supposed to have been, a sea of about 30-plus people turned the corner, launching anything they had at us. Bottles, sticks, you name it, they had it, and it was all being thrown our way. Never felt fear like it. As I ran back to the base and sat down to gather my breath, my inspector said, 'That was lucky team, we could have had another Keith Blakelock on our hands.' Keith Blakelock was a police officer who was murdered in the Broadwater Farm riot in Tottenham in 1985. As he fell, some 30–50 people surrounded him, and he was found with a six-inch-long knife in his neck, which killed him.

My feelings towards the job were never quite the same after that night. But when I had a panic attack on duty, I knew it was time to leave, which, although it was the right decision, brought its own set of complications. Being a police officer gave me a sense of status and identity. If I wasn't a police officer anymore, who was I?

I certainly wasn't myself for a number of months. I was stressed, drained and felt the most fragile I had ever felt. Two years after leaving, I am the happiest I've ever been. I stopped caring about what people thought of me, and I stopped worrying about how I would look to others, finally acknowledging that suffering in silence was a bad idea.

Now, if I have an anxious day, I know how to manage those feelings and I have people I can talk to.

Anonymous
I was fearful of everything

I feel that not addressing the trauma of an abusive relationship, the stress of over-achieving, the perfectionism required by my PhD course, and experiencing workplace bullying all contributed to my poor mental health.

I started hallucinating. I was having panic attacks so vivid that I thought I was bipolar. My doctor advised that I voluntarily section myself. A man touched me on the leg in a nightclub and I launched at him, was thrown out by the bouncers in tears, with no recollection of what had happened.

I went home to Glasgow. I have been to counselling, I'm taking medication (propranolol) and getting my confidence back. When I opened my laptop for my first freelance job on returning to Glasgow, I was fearful of everything.

I am now feeling like I am able to take on a job and not let it spiral out of control to the point where I have to quit. Things are getting back under control. I still have a bit to go when it comes to writing, but little steps like redoing my CV have led to public speaking, to making new friends on my course, signing up to university societies, getting involved, and to running new events.

All of these things are what give me life and what I enjoy doing. When it comes to mental health, how you recognise and protect your boundaries is so important.

4

My Shit Meds

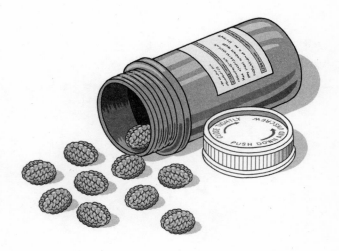

FOUR YEARS AGO, I BEGAN TAKING ANTIDEPRESSANTS for the first time. It was about 18 months after my first major depressive episode, and I still wasn't right. I'd tried counselling, I was eating well – during one particularly bleak episode I'd even started running – but this still wasn't enough to keep my depression at bay. It was time to consider medication.

I went to see my GP and asked for something to 'take the edge off'. I thought I could take a little helper as and when I needed it. Feeling anxious? Just pop a little pill, and POOF. No more mads.

But no. While that's a crude analogy for how some anti-anxiety medications work (like diazepam, for example), those types of medication are generally prescribed for a short period. I needed something more long-term, which I'd take every day for a cumulative effect. My GP recommended an SSRI (selective serotonin reuptake inhibitor) that I'd have to take every day for up to three weeks before they had an effect. By that time, I was so desperate for something, anything, that I agreed to start on 10mg a day of citalopram. I got my prescription and marched straight from the surgery to the chemist. While starting a chemical-altering medication doesn't necessarily call for celebration, I was optimistic, almost excited.

The first few days were monstrous.

I was working in the train station cafe at the time, which I had grown to love. It wasn't glamorous and I started most days at 6am, but I had a 30-second commute from my flat, the pay wasn't that much lower than what I'd been on at the comedy company, and I was finished by 2pm, which gave me time and energy to write my blog.

The cafe was always full of mums with prams, dog walkers

and hungover visitors desperate to smother their despair with chunks of sourdough bread and bacon fat.

I'd been taking the medication for about three days, with no ill effect, but one morning I felt... *wrong*. It's hard to describe. There was no nausea, no headache, no physical symptoms at all. It simply felt like someone had turned up the volume and brightness of the world. Everything felt close, and loud, and my movements were slow and clumsy. I spilt a 3kg bag of ice which scattered across the kitchen floor. I broke a mug. I mis-poured coffee beans into the grinder and sent them racing across the worktop. I cut my fingers. I didn't eat. I barely spoke as I doggedly arranged and rearranged cans of Perrier and cartons of coconut water. I drank herbal tea (the phrase 'herbal tea' pisses me off as well. All tea is herbal. Tea is a herb. Don't @ me). Depression is the most horribly isolating thing, a smudged screen between me and the world. I couldn't quite meet the eyes of my colleagues or customers, so I chained myself to the coffee machine, where I spent my shift steaming milk and grinding beans. I kept my eyes down, and cowered behind the enormous steel beast. Each stranger who approached the counter to collect their coffee was a threat, each cheery 'Thanks!' as I handed over each chai or Earl Grey or Americano was imbued with menace.

Finally, mercifully, my shift ended. I staggered home and climbed straight into bed, barely able to say a word to my long-suffering partner. I don't think I'd ever slept as much, or as badly, as I did over the next few weeks. I never felt rested, just varying levels of jangling anxiety.

When I'd been on meds for about four months, I slept through my 5:30am alarm. My boss rang me 20 minutes after

I should have been at work. I leapt out of bed, ran to the cafe, apologised, set up and was ready and open for my first customers by 6:30am. Six hours later, at the end of my shift, it occurred to me – I hadn't thought about my morning once. In the past, I would have torn strips off myself for making such a stupid mistake. But not that day. It had happened. I'd apologised to my boss, who was fine with it. And I'd got on with my day, without second-, third-, fourth-guessing every decision I made.

That's the difference the drugs make. They reduce the anxiety, so that you can get on with your life without a constant assault of intrusive, worrying thoughts. And they still do, for me.

That's not to say that I'll be on drugs forever. I might be, of course, but that's not a decision I have to make right now. And the truth is, I'm terrified of the withdrawal if and when I do stop taking them.

After I'd been on medication for three years, I ran out of pills. I kept meaning to reorder, but when I realised I was down to the last handful it occurred to me that I could just... *not* reorder them. See how I coped without them. I'd been having nagging doubts about whether or not I *really* needed them, whether or not they were a placebo, a crutch, and whether they might actually be a barrier to my full recovery from my mental illness. What if I was becoming reliant on medication I didn't need? I was feeling so much better than I had when I started taking them. I'd made massive structural changes in my life to remove what I perceived as the cause of my depression, while the medication helped me manage the symptoms. I wasn't stressed about work. I'd moved from London to Bristol – its friendlier, more chilled-out cousin in the West Country. I was exercising and eating fairly well. I was aware of my triggers and had a fairly good idea of how to look after my mental health. Naturally, I didn't want to take medication if I didn't need to. And I couldn't find out whether or not I needed it without doing without it for a while. Maybe now was the right time to try that. So without going to see my GP to get medical advice, I eked the pills out, tapering off to half a pill every other day, then nothing.

Very soon, this proved to be a terrible idea. A really dangerous, stupid, ill-informed, uncontrolled decision that was a threat to my stability and safety. Please, please don't stop taking your meds without medical supervision, like I did. I was a naughty idiot. Always speak to your doctor first.

Marian Keyes once said it's a sorrowful thing when the painkillers are taken away. How true.

The first week without medication was a horror show. Withdrawal impacted my spatial awareness – I'd often misjudge my step and walk into door frames, and my movements felt dopey and cumbersome. At my pub job, I pulled pints seemingly in slow motion, and always, always overpoured. I'd walk the floor, collecting glasses, serving food, feeling like a ghost, floating just a few inches outside my body. I put down plates extremely slowly to make sure that I didn't miss the table. There was a lot of tripping up over my suddenly-too-big feet.

I've since learned that this feeling of being disconnected from your body is called dissociation, and it's usually associated with profound trauma. Which I haven't endured. I'm just lucky, I guess.

A week later I was in the passenger seat of my boyfriend's car. Traffic was heavy – rush hour on a white-hot Saturday, and day-trippers were returning from the beaches of Portishead and Weston-super-Mare and Clevedon to the beer gardens of Bristol's city centre.

The temperature soared in the late afternoon sun. I felt feverish and nauseous. Anxiety began to writhe in my belly.

As soon as the word 'panic' fluttered into my consciousness, the attack was upon me.

I seized up in my seat as my adrenaline surged. Every working component of my brain was overloaded and overwhelmed, everything felt *bigger* and *louder* and *closer* and *more dangerous* than it had seconds before.

A car in the opposite lane appeared to lurch into ours before passing us by. So did the next one. And the next. And the next. In my skewed and anxious state, it seemed that every single car that passed was careering towards us.

I begged my boyfriend to stop the car.

'I can't,' he said, pained. 'There's nowhere to stop.'

We can't have been doing more than 50 in a 60-miles-per hour zone, but it felt like we were on black ice, out of control, speeding towards certain death.

For 40 agonising minutes, I crawled inside my skin, flinching as hundreds of tonnes of metal skimmed passed us.

And yes, logically, rationally, I *knew* that there was no threat. But my powerful irrational brain *believed* that there was, and that disconnection made me feel like I was insane.

Eventually, my bewildered man pulled over in a residential area marked by the vibrant street art that makes Bristol the city it is. I loved, and still love, the painted streets of my adopted home city, but today the acid-laced swirls and violent slashes of colour elevated my unease, and I cried myself breathless.

He didn't understand how I felt, although I know he tried to. How could he?

And how could I be anything but mad? It was a light, bright, beautiful day, one of the handful that we get in the first summer of a new relationship, and I'd ruined it by being mental.

When the panic was over, I felt properly mortified at Being Mad in front of my boyfriend. I didn't mind *telling* him about my depression or my anxiety, but showing him? Actually revealing to him how much my dickhead brain could hurt me? That was just too much. I felt vulnerable and embarrassed, and was certain he'd go off me. And as much as I'd love to say otherwise, I'm pretty sure he did go off me after that.

* * *

Later on, I curled up on my bed.

Two weeks without meds, I said languidly to myself. *Surely, this has to be as bad as it gets. Surely the withdrawal must be coming to a close.*

The next day I decided that going for a run might be a good idea. Endorphins, fresh air, that good ache in your thighs when you know you've worked your muscles. I set off on my new favourite route, through the allotment, past the eco-friendly houses that look like the cottages in the Shire, up into the woodlands. I hadn't run for a couple of weeks, so I took things slow and steady. I strolled uphill, stopped for a moment to take in the view of the city farm and the abundant veggie patches, then trotted along to the park with the heart-shaped lake.

I kept my pace gentle, but I was making enough impact to lose my breath a little.

It felt good.

Until it didn't.

Until it felt like my lungs had detached, and like I was drowning in too-dry air that I couldn't process.

Then my heart rate shot up.

And my brain started talking to me.

In this scene Michelle is played by Jodie Whittaker. Brain is played by Mark Heap.

EXT. BRISTOL STREET.

                    BRAIN

You're getting out of breath.

                    MICHELLE

That's OK. Exercise is meant to make you
lose your breath. It's all good

                    BRAIN

Yeah, but your heart's beating really fast,
too. Is that normal? I don't think that's
normal.

                    MICHELLE

Mate, we're running. Blood's got to pump,
lungs have got to breathe. It's all good.

                    BRAIN

But what if you're having a panic attack,
though?

MICHELLE

I'm not having a panic attack.

BRAIN

But what if you're having a panic attack?

MICHELLE

I'm not having a panic attack. I'm just doing exercise.

BRAIN

Well, the signs are there and it feels like a panic attack, so I think it's got to be a panic attack. I'm sounding the alarm.

BRAIN proceeds to trigger a panic attack. Foghorn sounds, red and yellow lights flash, neurons charge around screaming 'save yourselves!'

MICHELLE

(shouting)

No! Calm down! These signs are endorphins, remember? They're not going to hurt us!

BRAIN

(shouts back)

I hate endorphins! I say it's a panic attack, so it's a panic attack! Now sit down on that park bench over there and cry until I say you can stop!

So I sat down on the bench. Nothing was going to make me leave the sanctuary of this bench. The bench was a safe space.

People strolled by – dog walkers and families with young children in buggies. I waved away any concerned looks with a watery smile – I didn't need anyone to be nice to me, sympathy would only make me cry more. I phoned my local surgery, and was put through to the triage doctor immediately.

'I came off my medication two weeks ago,' I explained snottily. 'And I still feel awful.'

I explained what I'd done and what had happened. It's embarrassing, trying to talk about something very private in a public place while you're hyperventilating. But she was very calming and very kind, and suggested the single most helpful thing that would make me feel better.

'OK,' she said. 'How would you feel about going back on the medication?'

'Oh God, yes please,' I begged, weak with gratitude.

'I think that's a good idea. Your prescription will be ready in a couple of hours.'

* * *

After a few days back on the meds, I felt my crooked brain click neatly back into place. I felt my floating-ghost self align with my physical self – no more bumping into door frames, no more spilling pints. I felt 'right' again.

Recent studies have shown that the drugs *do* work – antidepressants are more effective than a placebo. But even if these studies had been inconclusive, I think I'd still take them. If, when I became ill, I could have taken six months off work and immediately started talking therapy on the NHS, if I lived in a culture where mental health was given the same priority as physical health, would I have had a breakdown? Would I have needed to take medication? Perhaps not. But opting out of work, of earning, of paying bills, of socialising, of *living your life* for months and months simply isn't possible for most people. So how else do we navigate life when we're not managing?

Sometimes I'll see an old picture of myself and spot something painful behind my eyes and think, *That looks like a mad person*. Mental illness feels to me like a loss of the self. If everything you care about, everything you love and value, no longer feels meaningful to you, what is life for?

The truth is that even if I never fall properly ill again, there will always be a part of me that fears Going Mad (and please, universe, if you're reading this, don't let me go mad again. Let me break every bone in my hands and feet, but please don't touch my brain). I don't feel truly in control of my brain and I know that it could throw a major wobbly at any point in the future. So to minimise the likelihood of this happening, I keep taking the meds.

I also try and keep tabs on my triggers. Yours might be different, but here are a few of the most common.

Triggers to be aware of

Hunger

I had fainting spells when I was a teenager, due to low blood pressure. I now know that if I don't eat within a couple of hours of waking up, I'm a mess. It's partly psychological – I worry that if I don't eat, I'll faint. But it's also, obviously, a real, strong physical response to hunger. I don't just get hangry, I get anxious, tearful, and panicky.

Alcohol

Even a single glass of wine is enough to disrupt my sleep, which will make me twitchy the next day. I do drink, but I try not to as a habit – if I don't really fancy booze, I'll stick with non-alcoholic beer.

Change

Change doesn't come naturally to me. The part of me that dearly wants to settle down, have one steady job that I like, build a home, get a dog, is horribly at odds with the me that wants to try everything once, tick off experiences like making a podcast, doing a photoshoot with a friend, travelling and writing a book. So almost against my instincts, I make myself go beyond my regular day job. Each new project brings joy, but it also brings uncertainty and anxiety, and I know I need to manage that.

Menopause

Most women experience a monthly hormonal cycle for between 30 and 40 years. When that cycle changes, of course it's going to affect your mood in some way.

Moving house

It's up there with death and divorce.

Clothes

Trying on clothes in mirrored changing rooms makes me feel deeply uncomfortable. I'm quite happy with my body. I enjoy it. I don't think about it a lot. It's a vessel. But there's something about being confronted by other people's ideas of my size and my body – that is, the ideas of whatever brand I'm trying on – that I find very unsettling. One trick that helps me is to turn away from the mirror and gauge how the clothes feel before I consider how they look. Does the fabric feel nice? Can I sit down and move comfortably? That's what's important, and often, it's the clothes that you feel secure, comfortable and confident in that make you look your best.

Changing seasons

Over the last couple of years I've noticed a tangible downturn in my mental health around the time the clocks change. I feel my energy levels flatten, and I sleep more. Perhaps my mammalian body gets confused when the hot yellow thing in the sky stops showing up so often. I'm now much more prepared for a seasonal low patch. Around the time of the change from winter to spring, and from autumn to winter, I'll keep a closer eye on my mood, my diet and my sleeping patterns. I'll make low-pressure plans with friends – a coffee, or a Skype session in my pyjamas – to prevent me from feeling isolated. I'll run until my breath is ragged and my muscles burn, so that when I'm in the shower afterwards I can close my eyes and listen to my blood play its stubborn beat.

I accept that my brain will behave like an utter shit three or four times a year. I'd like to think that it might stop, but it might not. So, like I said, I take the meds.

What are you on?

The northern seaside town of Blackpool – a beacon of British comedy and culture – has the highest rate of antidepressant use in the UK, with one in ten adults using meds to manage their mental health. So I decided to head up to the Las Vegas of the North to chat to some people about their experiences.

I have a deep affection for off-season tourist traps, probably because my home town is one. 'Faded glamour' is an unavoidable cliché in Blackpool, where butchers' shops and old-school tea rooms jostle shoulder-to-shoulder with casinos, clubs and tarot readers. Frank Sinatra played here three times in the 50s, in front of delighted crowds of restauranteurs, fairground staff and teachers.

I arrived around midday on a bright October morning. I'd posted my plans on Instagram – I had made a sign that read I TAKE 20MG OF CITALOPRAM A DAY FOR ANXIETY AND DEPRESSION. WHAT ARE YOU ON? – and explained I would carry it to the Pleasure Beach theme park. I received dozens of messages of support from all over the world. Bolstered by this, I imagined a steady stream of fellow sufferers making themselves known to me, coming over for a long chinwag about their experiences.

The moment I arrived in the town centre I knew I'd made a mistake. Yes, the conversation about mental health is ongoing, yes, people are writing books and tweeting and going to meetings and being a lot more open about how they really feel, but do they really want to talk to a stranger about it? Would people want to identify themselves as medication users, never mind share their personal story on a cold Sunday in October?

Expectations suitably lowered, I headed for Blackpool Central Pier, where I sat with my clearly visible sign propped up next to me. I made notes in my book, while furtively looking up at passers-by to see whether there was any interest, any curiosity at all.

The best I could hope for was that someone would see the sign and strike up a conversation. That was my plan. It was a deeply, deeply flawed plan, but it was the best I had. My project felt doomed, but I had to give it a try anyway. I was exposing myself, properly, live, in the flesh, as a mad person – quite literally signposting my madness. I felt alone, lonely and embarrassed. Old-time music hall tunes flooded from the nearby cafe. People were here for a bracing walk along the pier, to eat fish and chips and go home, not to talk about their mental health – or more specifically, the medication they used to treat their mental health. I was asking entirely too much.

I felt like shit. I didn't feel empowered. I wasn't reclaiming my narrative, I was being an arse, imposing my story on people who frankly weren't interested in it.

So I listened to the sea and watched dogs race across the shoreline. A steady stream of families wrangling boisterous kids, cuddled-up couples and adult children with their elderly parents passed me by, without so much as a look.

A regal-looking woman in her late 50s strolled past. She cast her eye over the sign and her mouth twitched in a smile.

She glided over to me with her hand outstretched. 'I'm on sertraline. It's saved my life.'

I stood and shook her hand, smiling through the lump in my throat. She'd seen me, and she'd let me see her. She seemed to read my mind and touched my cheek.

'Thank you. You're doing a wonderful thing.'

She embraced me, then moved on. I sat back down and allowed myself a short, happy cry.

A few minutes later I heard a young mum gasp, and she turned to her own mother and exclaimed: 'Mam! Look! That's what YOU'RE on!'

I waved, and they waved back. They gestured at the three small boys rolling and rioting at their feet.

'Can't stop,' the mum called. 'But thank you.' She gave me a quick thumbs-up and returned to wrangling her raging grandchildren.

A nervous, impeccably dressed older gentleman who sounded exactly like Alan Bennett took off his cap when he approached me and said, 'I have the same complaint.' We had a brief chat, then shook hands, and he went about his day.

OK, my experiment didn't have a far-reaching real-life impact that day, but I hope the few people I chatted to felt seen and validated by someone publicly 'outing' themselves as a medication user. And from the comments on my posts, my efforts left a few people feeling more empowered to have difficult conversations about their mental health and their medication use.

But you don't need to announce it to the whole world like I did if you don't want to. As long as you know that using whatever medication you need to stay healthy isn't shameful, you're doing all right.

* * *

How has taking medication affected your mental health?

Harald
It was like a David Lynch film

When I finally admitted that I have a serious mental health issue, I started to take antidepressants. Where I'm from you get prescribed enough for a month, then you have to visit a psychiatrist to reorder it.

Imagine this. It was like a David Lynch film. You enter a small room, and there's a desk cluttered with papers. In a very old high leather office chair sits a guy with dark hair and little round glasses. He barely looks up. Behind him is a huge metal cabinet, filled with different boxes of pills. He asks, 'How do you feel?' You mumble, 'OK,' and you get your pills for another month. You do this for six months and then you ask, 'When will we start the therapy? Do I have to take the pills for the rest of my life?' He says, 'Yes. Aren't you feeling better?'

That day, I left and looked for another doctor.

Holly
I used to be ashamed of my meds, but after four years
I'm happy and talk openly about my experience

My GP recommended antidepressants and counselling, as apparently they work best hand in hand.

I refused the meds that time, as I felt weird about it and didn't want to take them. I waited and waited to be referred to a counsellor, but in that time things got worse. I couldn't cope.

So I ended up on the meds, 50mg of sertraline. And wow, I felt great! Like, super-great! Like WOW!

The next two years were fantastic, I started running, went on holiday, got a fab new job.

I used to be ashamed of my meds, but after four years I'm happy and talk openly about my experiences. For me, they changed my life. I feel like they make me the me I really am. I treat them much like the contraceptive pill now, or my hay fever tablets.

Rachel

It has saved my life

I've been dealing with panic attacks for about seven years now, and although I've talked to several therapists, I've never figured out why it's happening and how I can stop it. I've tried mindfulness and listening to a 'calming' voice on a recording during my attacks, neither of which helped me much. My next therapist told me I needed to accept what's happening to me. She said I should just 'go do things that scare you: exposure, exposure!', so I went on a study trip to Portugal and had the worst three nights of my life before flying back early because I was so exhausted from not sleeping. And after a while, she concluded she couldn't help me and we had to part ways, because I didn't want to 'go outside for a walk and get distracted' when I was in full panic mode (I can practically only scream and cry on my bed when I'm in full panic mode, but sure, I'll take a nice walk around the neighbourhood).

Then I broke up with my husband, which caused such bad panic attacks that I was afraid to leave the house, couldn't eat without throwing up and couldn't sleep. Finally, I went to the doctor and asked for medication. Luckily, the psychiatrist took me seriously and put me on 10mg of escitalopram [an antidepressant] and 10mg of oxazepam [a sedative] for direct relief during a panic attack. It has saved my life. I can go out – even eat out again. I can meet up with friends. And I got myself a new therapist, who takes me seriously.

Pete

I wish I'd stopped taking the pills sooner

I went off sick from work and gained a CPN [community psychiatric nurse] who would visit me twice weekly.

I got a therapist who was totally useless and told me there was nothing wrong. I complained, and finally got a therapist who helped me. Besides being overworked in a high-stress job and in an abusive relationship, I'd never had the mechanisms to deal with the trauma of finding my great-grandad dead in bed when I was only three, and then finding my grandad dead a year later.

By this point I had two young children, but the medication left me feeling like a zombie and I was still in the abusive relationship. I tried stopping my meds but had severe withdrawal symptoms, so started taking them again. I spoke to my therapist and explained my intentions, and she agreed to monitor me, in case I went off my trolley. Over a month or two I reduced my dosage until I was completely off the medication. When I'd started to get my life in order, my abusive partner left me with my children.

I still have days when I feel depressed, but I have come to embrace my illness as part of who I am. My head is clear and sharp now. I have been medication-free for over ten years. I wish I'd stopped taking the pills sooner because I feel I missed my children's first few years, but it's all been worth it for having them now.

Nicholas
I have spent over half my life medicated

Now 32, I have spent over half my life medicated, while also not taking my mental health seriously. During those 17 years I have stopped (cold turkey) taking my meds (many different kinds and brands and dosages), more times than I can remember. The last time I did this three years ago, I destroyed a relationship, fucked up professional commitments, stopped paying my rent and bills and set myself on a path that a year later would result in the worst breakdown I have experienced.

Anthony
I've learned to take things one day at a time

I take:
Fluoxetine [Prozac]: 20mg in the morning.
Amlodipine [for high blood pressure]: 20mg in the morning.
Quetiapine [an anti-psychotic]: 300mg at night.
Atorvastatin [to lower cholesterol and prevent heart disease]: 10mg at night.

I'm 45. I was physically attacked twice within a 12-month period in 2012, which caused me to have a depressive episode. I was in a really bad place and went to hospital three times, because I was not coping with life. I still have thoughts that I'm better off not being here, but I've learned to take things one day at a time. I was also diagnosed with PTSD, for which I'm having treatment at present, including EMDR (eye movement desensitisation and reprocessing). I'm not sure how it works, but it is working.

Erica

I shed layers of hostility like clothing, each layer freeing me

I had been on quetiapine for almost five years. Worst decision ever. It literally turned me into an angry, hostile, difficult person. I lost myself. The meds exhausted me, changed my personality, made me angry, made me a zombie.

It took a horrific fight with my husband and being literally days away from divorce before I realised who I really am.

One choice led to another, then another. I shed layers of hostility like clothing, each layer freeing me. I stopped taking that horrible drug. I thought about who I was, who I wanted to be. I snapped out of the drug-induced haze and I discovered how to heal, how to embrace my body, how to love myself again. I fell in love with the girl I used to be and let her come out again. I grew thankful for my husband, our children, our grandchildren, our life. I found my voice. I spent hours talking to my husband and got the man I fell in love with back. We have a beautiful life. I'm thankful for everything my crazy, screwed-up past gave me. I'm grateful for my mental health.

I wish I'd had this epiphany way earlier. Unfortunately, society places stigmas on mental health, you're judged if you don't fit into its version of normal. Because of that, I just kept forcing pills down. Now I can communicate and voice how I want to be treated, without fear.

5

My Shit Therapist

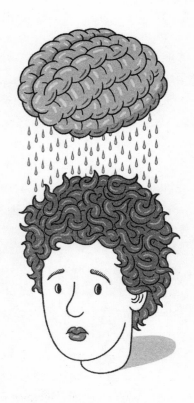

AFTER I FIRST WENT MAD, WHEN I WAS SO ILL I QUIT MY JOB with the comedy company, I knew I wasn't experiencing a proportionate, natural response to life's ups and downs, but severe clinical depression. Even so, I tried to fix it myself:

I ate well.

I ran.

Eventually, I tried medication.

And I saw a shit therapist.

My GP had given me the name of an NHS-recommended counselling service. It took such a Herculean effort to contact them, arrange an appointment and work out the best route from my flat to the clinic that the moment I put the phone down after calling them I went to bed, shattered.

I washed and dressed myself. I wore a black skirt and a lurid 80s print shirt. 'You look like a children's TV presenter, like Timmy Mallett,' my sister lamented.

'If I die before you do, you have to wear it to my funeral,' I retorted.

My bleached hair splayed like dead straw from under an ugly hat. I surveyed myself grimly in the mirror – a pale, tired, fret-lined face between Warhol-white hair, and a shirt that looked like a panic attack.

I traversed South London – a 20-minute walk to the train station, 25 minutes on the train, then a 15-minute walk to the clinic. A marathon, in my mind.

I was assessed in a beige room by a woman who looked like a discount Karren Brady – skirt suit, swishy hair, unflinching gaze. I told her how bad I felt. She surveyed me, talking me through a list of symptoms on a clipboard, literally ticking boxes as she read each one in a bored-sounding monotone.

'Have you been in despair for two weeks or longer?'

'Yes,' I said, my eyes darting around the room, desperate for something to focus on. Window. Box of off-brand tissues. Ugly plastic flowers. Window again.

'Have you thought about death?'

'Yes,' I said.

'Have you thought about hurting yourself?'

'No.'

'Have you thought about hurting your partner?'

'*No!*'

I couldn't bear the thought of the man I loved being in pain. That was another thought that kept me awake, filled me with fear all day, every day. He worked in Camden, where a few weeks earlier a man had been killed by a falling shop sign in a freak accident. I was convinced that something equally horrifying might happen to him. It was all I could do to stop myself from weeping as he left in the morning for work. Sometimes I couldn't even do that.

'No, I never imagine hurting my partner.'

She nodded with satisfaction and made another mark on her assessment sheet.

'Each session will cost £20,' she said.

'Oh,' I faltered.

I'd just quit my job. On the clinic's website, it had said that they'd make allowances for people on low incomes, charging £1 for every £1,000 they earned in a year.

'Is there any flexibility at all there?' I asked timidly.

'We'd need proof of income for that,' she sniffed.

'I don't have any.'

I didn't have any proof because I didn't have any income.

She fixed her eyes on me, flicked her luscious hair, and said nothing.

'OK, £20 is fine,' I conceded.

The doctor had told me that this would work, and I couldn't wait months for the entirely free service provided by the NHS. More importantly, I didn't have the strength to negotiate.

'When you get home, watch Brené Brown's TED talk on the power of vulnerability. It'll help,' she instructed me.

I went home, cried, and watched the TED talk. It was, and still is, excellent, but it wasn't the help I needed, the help that I had hoped my designated counsellor would be able to offer me, which suddenly seemed less likely.

* * *

At my first proper counselling session, I followed Lilly, a surprisingly grandmotherly figure, up the stairs to another low-lit beige room. I don't know why mental health professionals seem to think beige is a neutral, calming colour. It irks me. It's a very *smug* colour, I think.

And for the second time in my life, I gave voice to the unsayable things in my head.

There's a particular kind of despair that comes from hearing the thoughts that have been hurting you out loud.

Thoughts like:

I'm constantly afraid that something terrible is going to happen.
I'm terrified that my boyfriend will die.
I hate myself.

These thoughts, these words, have a particular shape and texture. They are familiar, yet frighteningly alien when you examine them outside the confines of your brain. Confronting them by saying them out loud in front of a stranger feels like skinning yourself alive. Acknowledging that you're mentally unwell, pulling back the curtain on your own mind and letting someone see the horrors in there for the first time, is the most naked, the most powerless, you'll ever feel.

During that first session, I cried for most of the hour. I told Lilly I cried all day, most days. I told her about my sudden aversion to loud noises, my spatial sensitivity (even supermarket trolleys seemed... *sinister*, like sentient steel animals, gliding malevolently in my peripheral vision as I did my weekly shop). I told her about the constant leaden sense of impending doom.

She nodded and seemed to agree with me a lot.

I didn't begin to relax or feel safe, but as I let out the poison that had been colouring my life over the last six months, like shit-tinted spectacles, a new feeling – relief? Liberation? The onset of mania? Who knows – stole over me.

'What does it feel like when you're having a panic attack?' she asked.

So I told her.

What does it feel like when you're having a panic attack?

It's like a migraine in your chest.

Like a wasp nest in your windpipe.

Like no one can help, because no one knows what's wrong.

A kind stranger might loosen your scarf, or hold your hand, or bring you a chair, but all that means is that you'll die sitting down.

They'll call an ambulance, because when you clutch your chest, they'll think you're having a heart attack.

After I quit my job, every second I wasn't catatonic with depression I'd spend hustling for casual jobs. Some jobs were lovely – my favourite was running writing workshops for a theatre company (especially when half of them were cancelled after I'd signed the contract, so they still had to pay me in full). What I desperately needed was a decent period of time off, but I didn't realise that at the time; and even if I had, there was no way I could afford not to work. Then I found a freelance gig with an arts collective in Dunstable, running community engagement workshops for a new festival. It was creatively fulfilling, but not demanding – odd days spaced out over a few weeks, so I never felt under unbearable pressure. In between, I'd do promotional work – turning up in supermarkets wearing a branded T-shirt and ugly black trousers to try and talk people into signing up for a loyalty card.

It was an early morning start on the Dunstable job, so the night before, the arts collective put me up in a pub opposite Dunstable Priory, the site where Henry VIII's marriage to Catherine of Aragon was annulled. The receptionist gleefully told me that there were underground tunnels between the priory and the tavern, so that Horny Henry could pop over between signing execution orders for a bit of slap and tickle with the bar wenches (not her exact words).

I was anxious about this job, and, you know, about life generally. And the thought of spending the night alone in an allegedly-haunted-as-fuck hotel, where I was at risk of being polter-bummed by an infamous royal wrong'un, did not alleviate my dread. I slept propped up on cushions, the overhead light at full beam, with my glasses on. Thankfully no polter-bumming occurred, but it was still a bumpy night. My brain just wouldn't shut up. Another crappy thing about anxiety is that no one tells you how utterly tedious it can be. I wanted to sit my brain down opposite me and say, 'You're right, everything's terrible, we fail at every single endeavour and some disastrous event is about to befall us. But can we please go to sleep now, and get back to conjuring horrific thoughts first thing in the morning?'

The next day was a feverish whirl of activity – writing and planning, running workshops in youth clubs and residential homes for the elderly, chatting to passers-by about what we were doing and trying to convince them to get involved, and talking on camera. I didn't stop for lunch because I didn't feel like I could ask to take a break. This wasn't anyone else's fault – it would have been absolutely fine for me to say, 'I'm going to sit down for half an hour and have a bite to eat,' but I kept plugging on because it felt like what I should do, until it was announced that everyone was going home.

At 5pm I was on the rush-hour train back to St Pancras Station. The carriage was overfull and overheated. I was hungry and exhausted from little sleep before a busy day in new surroundings with new people.

I started to feel a new kind of peculiar, a sort of... *shudder* in my mind. I was hyper-aware of my surroundings – I wasn't able to tune out other people's conversations. One man I couldn't see was booming away about GUTTING and PLUCKING a DEAD pheasant and I couldn't help but overhear, and my anxious mind homed in on the viscera and violence and painted nauseatingly vivid images, a flourish of bloodied bones and gizzards and feathers.

All sounds and sights and sensations were turned up, like the ident at the beginning of the IMAX. Everything was bigger and louder than me. I felt small and far away from myself.

When we finally pulled in to the station, I hurled myself off the train and staggered towards the Underground.

St Pancras is one of the biggest and busiest stations in the capital, because it's directly connected to King's Cross. I understand that it is an incredible feat of architecture if you're into that kind of thing, but to me it is a hateful hellscape, a labyrinthine leviathan of a station. It's always at least two-thirds full of bewildered tourists and ice-cold business folk, and there are more entrances and exits than there are in *The Complete Works* of Shakespeare.

Rushing away from the day-trippers and backpackers and the pheasant-botherer, I felt dreadful. I saw two policemen at the barrier and briefly wondered whether I should tell them I didn't feel well, but they frightened me (did they have guns? Is that why they made me feel uneasy? Maybe). I just wanted to get home, so I marched past them – head down, elbows ready to fight through the crowds.

But it was too late.

I sensed that the terrible event I'd predicted the night before was going to happen right now, here in St Pancras Station. It was out of my hands.

It's called a panic attack because it is an attack. Nothing is happening, and then *everything* is happening all at once. Your mind and body travel at warp speed from 'something's not quite right' to 'I feel like I'm going to die now'.

In the crowd, I spotted a high-vis vest, and I knew that meant safety. I lurched towards it and addressed the vest directly.

'Please help me, I—'

No more words. I doubled over, clutching my chest. My lungs were broken. My throat was closed. There was, simply, no more air. It was like I'd swallowed a balloon – my throat was sealed, and nothing could come in or out. I clawed at my throat, beat my chest with my fist and watched as the feet under the vest scuttled away. Someone led me to a chair and prised the bags I was still clutching from my fingers. I promptly folded in half at the waist.

I remember seeing a fine thread of drool dangling from my mouth as I choked for air.

'She's having a heart attack,' I heard someone say. I knew I was surrounded, but my vision had darkened and I could only see my own feet and legs.

I shook my head firmly – no, that wasn't it – but I was also clutching my chest, so I can appreciate that I was sending some very mixed signals.

Breath was coming now, but too much of it, *all* of it, completely out of my control, racing in and out of me so fast and so hard that I felt certain my lungs would burst like paper bags.

I spat out a single word: '*Panic.*'

The thread of drool broke free from my lip and splatted on to the floor at my feet. A kind man took my hand and held it for a very long time.

'That's all right,' he said. 'Take your time.'

I was still doubled over, my head near my knees. He was standing, holding my hand up near his chest. It must have looked like he was praying over me.

My breath was rolling like waves now. Still urgent, but softer, more rhythmic, less of an assault.

My peripheral vision came back. My bags were still beside me. The little crowd had dispersed, leaving the kindly hand-holding man, the station duty manager and the bewildered Polish cleaner whose high-vis vest had signalled safety in a storm. Tearfully I thanked them all, and the manager helped me carry my bags to a nearby cafe before returning to his office. There I called my boyfriend and asked him to come and help me get home. Shaking with hunger now, I paid £6 for a spelt scone that tasted like granite.

I wished I was dead.

'*That's* what a panic attack feels like,' I told Lilly, tearfully.

* * *

Retelling – reliving – that story hurt. Talking through tears when you can't get your breath, hurts. I felt lonelier and more desperate than I had ever done in my life. But surely this was all part of the process of recovery?

My new counsellor nodded sagely. 'Well,' she declaimed decisively, 'if that happens again you need to…'

Even through the fog of my despair, I listened attentively. This is what I was here for. This was the cure. Lilly would show me the way out of this nightmare and give me the helping hand I so badly needed.

'…have a cup of tea,'

OK…

'And you need to think about something else,' she finished.

Wait, what?

And then she said it. The single most devastating, most

119

inappropriate thing that anyone has ever said to me. Worse than any break-up, any row, anything my most dearly beloved or my greatest nemesis could ever say to me.

'Because, you know, there are plenty of people in this world who are far worse off than you.'

In a daze, I nodded as her words settled over my head like a shroud. What an agonising, bitter disappointment.

The next time you're about to have a panic attack, just… don't. Have you tried that?

Really? No way! If only I'd thought of this before I quit my job, ruined my career, terrified my parents and chose to become a burden to my partner!

I thanked her and handed over the cash, but a few days later I called the practice and cancelled my next session. I'd shared my deepest pain with Lilly, at a point in my life when I already felt like a conduit for all the hurt in the world. I was learning every day how I could accommodate more and more hurt, like an infinite game of Misery Tetris. ('Look, there's a little nook we can cram a bit more despair into!'). Her apparent dismissiveness annihilated me.

Common wisdom tells us that the first step on the road to recovery is to admit that we need help. And that's a very, very hard step to take. So we invest a lot in the people we take that step with. We imbue doctors, therapists and counsellors with superhuman intuition. We assume that they've all had the same level of advanced and detailed clinical training for every possible scenario our shitty brains can throw at them. We desperately believe that their resources are limitless. That they never make mistakes. That they can fix us.

So when they fail to meet these impossibly high standards,

it's crushing at best. At worst, it's downright dangerous. While it's good to talk, it really, *really* matters who you're talking to. Because in such a vulnerable state, listening to the wrong person can be very bad for you indeed.

Crisis talks

It's Saturday and I'm diligently scribbling away at Bristol Central Library. There are a few of us dotted about – students, older people researching their ancestors (*Don't get too excited*, I think, uncharitably; *they were probably slave owners*), people holding work meetings. I'm wearing my clunky do-not-disturb headphones. I'm not actually listening to anything; I find music too distracting. I am, miraculously, both relaxed and focused on my prose. It's going well – fully formed paragraphs are emerging from my thoughts in a steady stream, and the word count is mounting up nicely.

Suddenly a low, rasping man's voice breaks the silence, making an unrepeatable threat in my left ear. I shriek, startled, tear off my headphones and jump out of my seat, spinning to face my assailant. For a microsecond, I think it must be a friend pranking me, and I burn with anger and shame and fear all at once.

There's no one there.

There's nothing but the shocked responses of the fellow library users and the staff all around. Everyone is staring at me.

'Who was that?' I demand of the room at large. 'Did you hear that?'

Silence. A few shaking heads.

'I heard a… it sounded like a voice saying—'

I stop myself. These people are already on their guard and I don't need to persecute myself further by telling them what I thought I'd heard. What I *had* heard. Hadn't I? Terror and distress mounted in my mind as it dawned on me that I was experiencing a new kind of mental dysfunction. The ugly name of a misunderstood-but-most-feared disorder – *psychosis* – flashed briefly behind my eyes. But I still had the insight to know that I didn't want to *seem* mad, even though it was probably far too late for this particular audience to reach a different conclusion.

'Jesus *Christ*,' huffed a woman behind me, who looked thoroughly pissed off at the interruption to her work meeting.

'There must be something wrong with my headphones,' I lied, trying to keep my voice even. 'I'm so sorry, everybody.'

'You must have been concentrating very hard,' said the library assistant, who was smiling at me with a gentleness that I'll always be grateful for.

My heart was death-dropping in my chest. I returned to my seat and tried to settle down to writing again, but it was no use. And in fairness, if there's a way of recovering your cool when you've just screamed at the top of your lungs in a public library and reared back like an elephant that's just seen a mouse in a vintage cartoon, I don't know of it. So I packed away my laptop and left. The moment I was outside in the fresh air I leaned against the library wall and cried like my heart was breaking. Like my brain was breaking.

Then I went home and looked into whether or not I needed to get myself sectioned.

* * *

'Hello, mental health switchboard?'

'Hi, my name's Michelle Thomas and I'm having a mental health crisis.'

'Righto,' came the inappropriately cheery, unfazed reply. 'My name's Ken. Why don't you tell me what's going on?'

His kindly Bristolian burr broke my heart.

'I was in the library. I... I heard a voice. That's never happened before.'

There was a pause. He seemed to perk up a bit. Maybe it had been a slow morning.

'Right. Are you safe? Are you worried you might harm yourself or anyone else?'

'Yes. I mean, no, I won't.'

'Oh, right, OK.'

Then he was silent. He almost sounded a bit disappointed. Clearly I'd exhausted his repertoire. I needed specific, clinical care. I needed to speak to someone who knew what they were dealing with and could offer me practical help. All he could offer was empathy and compassion. And empathy and compassion are wonderful, but they're not a clinical strategy for wellness.

'If you like, you could ring 111 and see if they could help? Or you could go to A&E?'

'Oh,' I said.

I was afraid of going to hospital. I didn't think I needed to be sectioned – I had enough insight to know that the voice wasn't real. I was frightened because it was happening, but I wasn't frightened of *it*. It was just a thing my brain was doing. But what could that mean? Bipolar, borderline personality disorder, schizophrenia... a litany of miserable diagnoses rattled through my head. *Please no*, I begged the God I don't believe in. I've got so much stuff to *do*. I've got *plans*. Books to write. Countries to visit. I want to build a home. To fall in love. I want to own a dog. I can't look after a dog if I go mental.

'Are you still with me?' Ken asked, less cheerfully now.

'Yes. Yes. Well, err… I'll see how I feel. Thanks.'

'OK. Well, would you like to speak to the women's switchboard? There might be someone there who can help?' He paused. 'They're for women' he emphasised, helpfully.

I took the number.

'Now, Michelle, I'm here until ten o'clock if you need someone to talk to. Just call me back, all right?'

'OK. Thank you.'

I called the women's crisis team. Unfortunately, I hadn't had the foresight to have a crisis during their working hours, so they couldn't help. I called 111. The operator there asked all the same questions, and arranged for a triage GP to call me back.

In the meantime, she gave me a different phone number for my local crisis team.

I called it.

'Oh… Hello again, Ken.'

I balled up on my bed, texted a few select friends to tell them what had happened, ordered a pizza, and spent the rest of the weekend huddled under a duvet, letting my loved ones' words comfort and reassure me while I waited for the GP to call me back.

The triage doctor finally called me back at 2:45am. It went to voicemail.

We need to talk about mental illness

We need to normalise mental illness, and eliminate stigma. This has been the bottom line for many of the most impactful and powerful mental health campaigns over the last five years. And yes, absolutely, couldn't agree more, double thumbs up to that message. But sometimes we – the ill – need to do more than talk. We need someone – a clinician, an expert – to explain to us what's going on, and what could happen next. I've been in crisis, and when that happens it feels like there's no middle ground between calling the Samaritans to cry on a friendly volunteer's shoulder, and taking myself to A&E, hoping I don't have to wait six hours for the psych team to assess me, and risking being sectioned against my will because I can't control and don't understand my brain's behaviour.

I know it's good to talk, I know it's important to talk, but I can't stress enough how much I didn't need to talk following that incident in Bristol Central Library. I needed someone to talk *to me*, to explain to me what had just happened. Someone to tell me whether or not I might have late-onset bipolar, or schizophrenia, or psychosis, and what that might mean; what causes auditory hallucinations and whether or not they're harmful. I needed to know whether I needed treatment and whether the symptom I had experienced could be corrected or cured, or just alleviated.

It's time to talk. Yes. But it's also time to properly fund vital mental health services. It's time to treat mental illness as the health crisis it is, not something that can be significantly improved with a cup of tea and a nice chat. Sometimes we need medical intervention.

There are so many well-meaning, non-clinical, volunteer-run spaces for those who need them. But with a lengthy waiting list for one-to-one counselling on the NHS in some regions of the UK, some sufferers on low incomes are not accessing the support they desperately need.

One woman told me that after she'd been raped, she contacted a counselling service. Her counsellor said that she'd only be able to treat her if she agreed to have their sessions recorded as part of a research project. The woman could barely articulate what she'd endured, and yet, at her most vulnerable, she was being asked to have the most painful experience of her life documented, filed, transcribed and pored over – not for her own benefit, but as part of someone else's coursework. She said she felt like a number.

I haven't experienced anything like the voice before or since. Aural hallucinations are listed as a possible side effect of my medication. It could have been stress. I've had blood tests and MRI scans on my brain, all of which came back normal. It might never happen again. It might be the first episode in a new kind of fun activity that my brain is engaging in. And unlike many who suffer from psychosis or schizophrenia, I know that the voice wasn't real. It was just a thing that my brain did – a brain fart, as a friend described it. It was distressing, but it was no more harmful to me than the depression and anxiety that I've already got a pretty decent handle on. So while I hope it doesn't happen again, I think I'll be all right if it does.

My actually-pretty-good therapist

What I didn't know when I first sought help is that there are many, many different kinds of therapists and counsellors: Gestalt therapists, humanistic therapists, Jungian therapists, psychoanalysts.

They can be expensive and difficult to access outside big cities. It can take planning, research and time – *so much* time – to find one that fits you. And when you're depressed and vulnerable, that's a formidable challenge.

A year or so after my disastrous first attempt at seeking help, I started getting psychotherapy.

And it changed my life.

Every Monday morning I arrived at Elaine's house – her actual home, which I always found odd. Why would she open her door to such chaos? She answered the door, gave me a kind smile and invited me to go upstairs ahead of her with a nod.

Her consulting room was bright. I took the same wicker chair and she sat opposite me next to a small table, where she put her glasses. Then she nodded, and I knew it was time to begin. For my first few sessions I'd ask how she was, how she'd spent her weekend, wasn't it a lovely/miserable day? Pleasantries over, I could cut to the main topic of conversation: me, me and me.

I've had therapy sessions where nothing interesting was said, by her or me. Whenever I tried to make her laugh, I rarely received more than a kind smile. I've had therapy sessions where I've gossiped about people I know and bored myself rigid, going on and on about the same petty perceived slights. I've had sessions where I've clutched my head, folded in on myself and wailed because I've had no idea how I'll manage to get through the monstrous marathon of agony that the day ahead holds for me.

I've had therapy sessions where I've made an absent-minded remark about an event from a decade ago that I've never told anyone about, then realised that barely a day has gone by when I haven't thought of it at least once.

I'd tell Elaine everything. And if nothing else, it was quite nice to go somewhere to talk about myself for an hour. It's extremely liberating to pay someone to listen to you be as selfish, boring, mean-spirited, unkind, angry, despairing and self-indulgent as you like, knowing that it's their job to *not* judge you. Making a space where you're allowed to explore the ugliest, saddest and most frightening parts of yourself is invaluable. I didn't have to worry about her feelings. I didn't have to be happy. Or funny. Or charming. Or interested in her at all, really. And as harsh as that sounds, when you're constantly consumed by thoughts about what a terrible bastard you are, it's a relief to pay to have that worry lifted from your shoulders for an hour.

It freed up so much space in my brain. If something happened to make me feel stressed or weird, just knowing that I had somewhere to dump those thoughts made me feel better. *I'll tell Elaine about that on Monday*, became my mantra. It soothed me.

I never missed a session. If I went on holiday or away for work, I'd Skype her.

Elaine rarely seemed to guide me in our sessions, or maybe she was an expert in making it look as if she didn't. She never formally began proceedings, and rarely asked questions. Every now and again she'd ask me to re-examine something

I'd said. One of the most useful things she did was repeat something I had said back to me, so that I could hear what I was truly thinking and feeling, and what prism I was viewing the world through.

There was a lot I didn't know.

I didn't know I was so cruel to myself.

I didn't know I had so much anger inside me.

I didn't know I cared so much about some event I was barely conscious of.

At the end of every session I felt better. There's a lot to be said for talking and not worrying about how it sounds. It's like going to a gym for your feelings.

There's that brilliant scene in *Black Books* where Manny and Bernard get therapy. Their therapist sits in stony silence and doesn't say a word, while they talk and talk until they unravel and come to their own perfect conclusion. Elaine was like that, but smilier.

At my first therapy session of the new year, I didn't ask if her Christmas was fun. I didn't ask her how her New Year's Eve had been. She answered the door with a smile and 'Good morning.' I walked into the consulting room. We sat down, then I talked about myself for an hour. I interrupted her occasionally, and I repeated myself, unloading a stream of consciousness *at* her, not *to* her. I rattled on and on and on and on and on.

At the end of it, she said, 'That's time, I'm afraid.'

She didn't say anything as I put on my coat. This was still a space where mine was the final word.

Then I said goodbye and headed to work.

God, it was lovely.

* * *

Some people thought it was very odd to have a therapy session at 8:30am on a Monday, but it set me up for the week. Afterwards, I'd walk to the bus stop and by the time my bus arrived, the session was far from my mind, and I was wondering what I would buy myself for breakfast, my weekly post-therapy treat.

Eventually, though, purging myself of my horrible thoughts stopped feeling useful. It started to get a bit boring. I felt that after a few months of brain-dumping, I was going around in circles. I wanted therapy to help me take control of my mind – I wanted feedback, strategies, exercises, homework. And she didn't give those to me because that wasn't her job. She's not that kind of therapist.

Seeing the 'wrong' kind of therapist for a year might seem like a mistake – and an expensive one at that – but it wasn't. She gave me what I needed for a while. The thing about therapy, of course, is that it isn't a magic bullet.

The received wisdom is that by talking about depression, by confronting it, you can free yourself of it, that when we admit we have a problem it is the first step to our recovery. Once we confront our demons, they are banished.

I regret to inform you, dear reader, that this is in fact horseshit. The pain abides. Of course it does. You can't out-talk it. Or out-think it. You can't reason with it. Or rationalise it. Or bore it away with one of those ten-minute meditation apps. Therapy isn't going to disconnect you from your pain. Unless you're disassociating (when you feel disconnected from the world or from yourself in some way), you're connected all the time. You live your discomfort every day.

When you start having therapy, you imagine dramatically

confronting your demons, screaming into the storm like Natalie Portman in *V for Vendetta*, then emerging purged, wiser, stronger. Happier.

But you don't. At least not until you've been at it for a few years. And even then, I imagine that finally understanding what makes you tick is a much quieter revelation. More of an 'Oh, I *seeeeee*' than a *Shawshank Redemption*-style escape to paradise.

It's that old assumption that we are either depressed or not depressed. Ill or well. Happy or sad. In fact, we are usually somewhere between the two.

How to choose your therapist

Ask around
You'd be surprised how many people you know are already in therapy. I chose Elaine by recommendation. Before I met her, I seriously considered basing my decision on Google Images. I had my eye on a woman with a reassuringly severe haircut – none of this layers and feathered textures nonsense, just a straight black no-bullshit bob. '*She'd* sort me out,' I thought approvingly.

Check their credentials
If you live in the UK, you can choose a therapist who's accredited by the UK Council for Psychotherapy or the British Association for Counselling and Psychotherapy. Their websites also have information on different kinds of therapy, so that you can consider what's right for you and check out the registered practitioners in your area.

Check your budget

The UK's NHS is amazing but it's criminally underfunded when it comes to mental health. I'm extremely lucky. When I started seeing Elaine I was working in a pub, and I wouldn't have been able to afford £45 for each weekly session. A very kind friend paid for me until I found a better-paid job.

Free services

In the UK, you need a GP referral for most mental health services on the NHS, but you can self-refer for some, like drug and alcohol services.

If you don't want to wait months for NHS treatment (and who does?) there are clinics where you can pay for treatment based on your income. And if you can't find what you need in your area, counselling apps and video chats with therapists are becoming increasingly popular.

Textcare from SANE is a wonderfully heartening and free service that provides support via a simple, calming text whenever you need it. The mental health charity Mind have compiled a list of apps, including their user forum Elefriends, that can help you manage and improve your moods.

* * *

Everyone's experience of talking therapy is different. How has therapy been for you?

Anonymous

My stay in hospital helped me get out of the rabbit hole

When the sick voice in my head tried to persuade me to swallow all the random pills in my medicine cabinet, when I got in the bathtub and wanted to drown, I knew this was a serious matter of life and death. I couldn't do that to my kids. I needed help.

My stay in hospital helped me get out of it again. My goal was to function. To eat, shower, to care about something. The people who were there with me saved my life. They all had big hearts, although they suffered from the same thing I did. They made me laugh, stop and look at the beautiful details of life. The therapy I received there gave me hope that one day I could feel normal again.

Holly

I call my therapist The Spoon

I chose my therapist because he said on his profile that he enjoyed juggling. It amused me. I couldn't imagine it. At my first therapy session I was a gibbering wreck. I was so flustered that I ended up misjudging my step and falling down 15 concrete steps in front of him before even introducing myself. My handbag flipped over my shoulder, spilling the contents all over the place.

I was still on the floor when I looked up and saw my therapist. 'Holly?' he said.

'Yes,' I said. 'I just fell down the stairs,' I added unnecessarily. He literally just stood there with his blank therapist face and didn't say a word. He didn't even acknowledge the accident, or ask if I was OK. So I picked myself up, gathered my belongings and hobbled after him, bleeding from a cut knee. That was my first session with the juggling therapist.

I had six sessions with him in total. There were lots of long, awkward silences. I felt like I hated him and told him so, but he didn't comment on it.

I stopped seeing him.

About four months later, one of 'my nights' happened. I wanted to cut myself so badly, but I already had two deep purple scars on my leg which I felt very self-conscious about. I ended up grabbing my long hair and cutting it off to chin length. Luckily it turned out OK, so I looked all right for work the next morning.

After that, I thought to myself, *You need better therapy, lady*. I was hesitant to start therapy again because of the cost. But I really felt like I owed it to my future self and decided to use my savings to pay for it, even though it meant eating noodles for tea.

Paying for therapy is awkward – should you hand over the money before or after the session? So I decided to go with putting the money in an envelope and handing it over straight away. It's hard not to feel a little like, 'Here's 60 quid, now you have to listen to me.' Then if he doesn't say anything useful enough, I feel cheated.

To this day I always dread the sessions – I think, *What the hell do I say today?* Funnily enough, these days end up being the most productive sessions. All sorts of shit comes out. I always leave feeling better.

I call my therapist The Spoon. There's this theory in

Buddhism. Imagine a glass of water. If you stir it with a spoon, sediment lifts up and clouds the water. The sediment is all your shit going on. And when something happens in life that we struggle with – a challenge, a break-up, it could be anything – that sediment is ours, and we're meant to thank the spoon for bringing it up for us to deal with. I'm not sure what I believe, but that's why I call him The Spoon.

Anthony

Talking is the best way to fight depression and anxiety

At university I had two episodes where I cut my wrists because I could not get my head around having dyslexia. I then came home because of my state of mind and took an overdose of paracetamol. I spent five days on a normal hospital ward to stabilise my body, then was discharged and just left to my own devices.

If I knew a man who was struggling with his mental health, I'd say to him first and foremost, don't let it fester too long and find someone to talk to about how you're feeling. Then you have to find a way of coping, without putting yourself or anyone else in danger. In my experience, talking is the best way to fight depression and anxiety.

Lauren

'You need to say that again, because it was very powerful.'

The worst thing a therapist ever said to me happened in marriage counselling with my dickhead-now-ex-husband. We'd shared that a big struggle in our relationship was my weight. I was eight weeks pregnant at the time, 180lbs [nearly

13 stone] at 5 feet 7 inches [170cm]. The therapist suggested I probably would benefit from weight loss because 'I' would feel so much better. 'Imagine carrying around a 20lb bag of flour and getting to set it down,' he said.

The best thing to come out of therapy happened a year and a half later, with a new therapist. I was telling her how fed up I was with my husband and with my life and so on. I said, 'I would rather live in a cardboard box with my daughter than spend another minute in that house with him.'

My therapist paused, looked directly at me and said, 'You need to say that again, because it was very powerful.'

No more words were needed. That was it. With the precision of a skilled surgeon, she cut away the bad and left the healthy tissue struggling to survive underneath to heal.

Claire

She suggested that this happened to me because
I trusted people too much

Oh, the stories I could tell, being someone who has been in and out of therapy all their life! However, I have to share the absolute SHITSHOW of an experience I endured after I went through rape. I was in the GUM [sexual health] clinic when I disclosed what had happened. I was literally forced into a room with a counsellor, after repeatedly saying that I didn't want to talk about it. We sat in silence. Every now and then they'd say, 'Do you want to talk about it?'

And I'd say, 'No.'

What a way to give a person their sense of control back.

A few months later I decided I was ready to talk, and I went to see a clinical psychologist. She suggested that this had happened to me because I trusted people too much and was too willing to share. This was based on my having told three close friends what had happened, and she felt this was too many. This conversation silenced me thereafter, because I felt like I shouldn't have been telling anyone about my sordid, dirty experience. I felt scarred for years until I began training to become a therapist myself, and learned that this psychologist was a very dangerous person who shouldn't have been in her position of power. I have since had so much positive therapy and my life has been a lot better.

Nicholas
*A therapist once told me I should have
sex with men*

A therapist once told me I should have sex with men. I thought she was a shit therapist at the time. I was very irritated, it almost felt like a schoolyard taunt. I felt angry that I was being dismissed. Two and a half years later I acknowledged that I was bi and came out, and felt much better.

Barry
I wanted one-to-one therapy

I've just started group therapy and I am struggling. It's the third session today and there are only six people in the group. One person has already left. I wanted one-to-one therapy but it's not available for me – I have asked and asked. I don't want to admit I am a victim, but explaining what is wrong with me makes me look like a victim.

James

*She said my mum had only wanted what
was best for me*

I didn't think I'd had an abusive upbringing until my 20s. The stuff I dealt with as a child was pretty common among my peers – Mum left Dad, took out her frustrations with Dad on us, remarried a violent asshole… I thought it was just a 'normal' childhood.

When I saw a therapist and told her about my relationship with my mum, I found her very dismissive. She said my mum had only wanted what was best for me. That pretty much killed the conversation, because I thought if my mum cared about my safety, I wouldn't have a chip of bone missing from my skull from being beaten, or a wonky jaw from my stepdad hitting me with a golf club.

I had a few therapists who were equally dismissive. It was almost as though me saying, 'My mum was bad', or, 'It was terrible having a stepdad' offended them and they'd shut down the conversation immediately. It's probably worth mentioning they were all female, and in all honesty, I wasn't entirely comfortable talking to a woman about how bad my mum was.

Sol

*He didn't show me the way, I found it,
but he gave me some direction*

I once paid £70 for 45 minutes, and he didn't even remember my name. I don't expect you to be my best friend but come on, check your notes before I get there.

A few years ago, I went to an addiction recovery place. You only get four sessions, and after I'd finished those they just palmed me off with someone new. She wanted to do sessions by video call, which felt way too impersonal.

I have a new therapist now. The price you pay depends on your income. He wears the same clothes, in the same room, on the same hour, every week. I'm curious, so I asked why. He said it's because some people need that level of routine to make them feel comfortable. And yes, I really feel very confident with him. I go every Friday, and it makes me feel good.

After 30 years of therapy, it's not like I go into each session and start crying, and that's that. I have to talk about my real feelings, show my real self, who I am. This is so difficult. And when it gets to this point in the sessions, normally I stop going. I start making excuses. When the thoughts are only in your mind, you can ignore them. But when you say them, they exist. They're real. There's a difference between discussing something that happened years and years ago, and something that's happening right now. And that's scary. For everyone, I think.

So, I go and cry, and there's this big catharsis. But once that's over I have to start putting the work in, and I run away. But when my son left home, I felt like shit. I texted my therapist and said I didn't want to go back, it was too much. My son's left because I'm not good enough. He's not a child anymore, he's an adult, and he can see my defects and that's why he's left. And that's so painful I can't talk about it.

My therapist said, 'I remember you told me a year ago in your first session, you always leave when it gets difficult. So, come for free to your last session, and say goodbye. You don't have to stay for the whole hour, you don't have to speak if you don't want to.' And after a lot of thinking, I went. I sat down in front of him and suddenly I couldn't stop crying. I didn't speak, I just cried. And he said, 'My door is always open for you.' I have to make the effort, not him. He just listens and gives me parameters so I can find my own answers. He didn't show me the way, I found it, but he gave me some direction.

6

My Shit Love Life

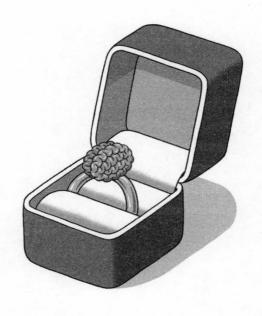

I FELL IN LOVE (BRIEFLY) A YEAR OR SO AGO. DURING THE heady initial stages of giddy limerence, I was very aware that my body was mistaking my racing heart and rising adrenaline for a red alert. Same physical symptoms, very different cause.

I was sceptical, cynical and scared. My heart said yes. My fanny said YES FUCKING PLEASE. My brain said... yeeees, BUT. BUT. A few weeks before I'd met this gorgeous creature, my brain told me I was going to die during a panic attack. It had told me I was the worst person in the world (objectively not true – I've never started a war or set fire to an orphanage or left a nasty book review on Goodreads), and that my parents would be better off if I'd never been born. How can you trust your brain when it's telling you you're in love, and that somebody loves you and that that's a good, safe, happy event, when it has proven itself time and again to be shiftier and less reliable than a Tory politician at a public debate about food banks?

Relationships terrify me, if I'm honest. I'm scared I'll be miserable, or that they'll be miserable and they'll be too polite to tell me. At least in the olden days if you took a risk and ended up in a loveless marriage, you'd be dead by 45. Looking for just one person who's going to make you happy for the next 50 years is a tall order. Marian Keyes wrote about this brilliantly in *The Break*, a novel about a couple who take six months apart and risk their marriage, because they're afraid of not doing everything they want to in this relatively short, brutal life.

It's the 'forever' thing, isn't it? That's what ruins everything. No one aspires to have a loving, fulfilling relationship for six, ten, fifteen years, and then call it a day while there's no ill will or resentment. It simply *has* to be until death do us part. What's that pressure doing to us?

And you don't just *acquire* a nice partner. You've got the arduous task of finding them, meeting them, spending time with them, talking to them, listening to them talk, going for meals you could cook at home and drinking alcohol when you don't really feel like it, because that's what people do on dates. It's exhausting and *terribly* unsexy. It feels like homework. You're trying to present your wittiest, prettiest, *least mental* self, while also trying to navigate secret codes of etiquette about dress, money, humour and physical contact so treacherous and so fraught with potential embarrassment that it's a wonder any of us leave the house, ever.

Online dating

I'm Michelle 😊
I'm a Taurus 🐃
I like long walks in the park 🌲
Powell and Pressburger films 🎬
and I'm taking citalopram for anxiety and depression 💊

Many of us share vast swathes of our lives online. For the last ten years, 25–35-year-olds have had the opportunity to present a 'best of' version of their lives. Millennials happily migrated from MySpace to Facebook and casually began to publicly document their lives in a way no generation had done before. Today, research by online dating site eHarmony suggests that in the near future, over 50 per cent of couples will meet online. Yes, *50 per cent*. So, as we post, OF COURSE we use the most flattering pictures we have. OF COURSE we want to seem like the coolest, smartest, funniest and best-looking version of ourselves. That's what we've trained ourselves to do, and that's what our social media role models do. We've created a world where when we can chat 24/7, create a profile that reads like a CV ('He likes Nordic Giants, too?! OMG, he's the one!') and send each other flattering nudes whenever the mood takes us.

It's a paradox. We are totally preoccupied by the way we represent ourselves online, all the while poring over others' yoga-on-a-beach profiles. We're afraid of the very thing we voraciously consume. What nourishes us also destroys us. What chance do we have of NOT going mad?

I believe this is corroding our ability to cultivate real emotional affinity. The one thing we can't create, fake and share online is intimacy. Familiarity based on sharing (or over-sharing) can be mistaken for it, but it's no substitute for the real thing. And when we do finally meet offline for the first time, we're so desperate for it to be there, we often see it when it's not. Humans have been running the getting-to-know-you gauntlet since time immemorial, but with online dating, we run it over and over and over again. That can put a tremendous amount of pressure on our mental health.

Nir Eyal, the author of *Hooked: How to Build Habit-Forming Products*, has spent several years consulting for the tech industry, and has terrifying insight into how the Silicon Valley giants operate. His research suggests that we have become truly, psychologically addicted to the technology we use every day, and it's no accident. Its designers had that in mind.

Have you ever been inside a casino? There are often no clocks and no windows, so you can lose all track of time. Lights keep you awake and alert. Garishly patterned carpets repel the eye to keep your head up and maintain your focus on the game. With dating apps, the same psychological hacks that keep us gambling and gaming are being used to hijack a fundamental biological imperative – to fall in love. Every time you swipe, you're getting a variable reward. Could be your soulmate. Could be an ad. Could be your dad. Research shows that 90 per cent of 18–29-year-olds go to sleep and wake up with their mobile phone. That's like keeping a one-armed bandit next to your bed.

The University of North Texas conducted research into the impact of Tinder on the mental health of over 1,300 participants. The results showed that users reported less psychosocial well-being than non-users. Particularly men. Men are three times more likely to swipe right, which means they're at greater risk of rejection and ghosting (when a romantic interest stops replying to messages). Both male and female Tinder users reported less satisfaction with their bodies and looks compared to non-users. It's also been found that 18–25 per cent of Tinder users are already in a relationship, and that non-single Tinder users score significantly lower on agreeableness and conscientiousness, and significantly higher on neuroticism and psychopathy compared to non-users who are in a committed relationship.

Research into the impact of online dating on mental health is sparse, but the proven impact of social media on mental health isn't promising. According to a study from the University of Pittsburgh, social media use is significantly associated with increased depression. Horrifyingly, it was recently revealed that Facebook has the capacity to identify when teenagers feel 'insecure', 'worthless' and 'in need of a confidence boost'. Advertisers could use this information to target users with any manner of products when they're at their lowest, from counselling apps to weight-loss supplements. How long before similar data is collected from our dating apps? And what will that do to our emotional wellbeing?

The thing that really impacts mood and well-being is the sense of time wasted. And when it comes to time wasted on dating apps, those feelings manifest as loneliness, isolation and a sense of worthlessness. The emotional labour we invest in endless messaging, making ourselves available at every waking hour without setting boundaries, and trying to make people like us is draining in itself, but when this doesn't pay off, it can be extremely damaging.

My generation is patient zero when it comes to the impact of social media and dating apps. There are no health recommendations for their use. I see it as being like the first heady years of the tobacco industry, when everyone looked sexy as fuck with cigarettes hanging between moist lips, oblivious to the havoc they were wreaking on their bodies. Only instead of lung cancer, the result could be profound psychological stress, emotional turmoil and repetitive strain injury in our thumbs.

How to use dating apps without going mental

1. Take some time over your profile.

    Choose your pics wisely – one selfie, one candid shot doing something you love, one full-length one that you're happy with, and one of you out and about with your mates to show how popular and well socialised you are.

    I've had messages from women who so fear being rejected at first sight, they've not only uploaded numerous full-length pictures from various angles, they've also graphically described their body shape to their dates in advance.

Of course, we need to be honest. We can't simply omit what will be apparent on a date. We need to post honest pictures of our *whole* selves, and if we knowingly misrepresent that, we're setting ourselves up for rejection. And why would we do that?

Listen to me.

You're ace.

I don't know you, but you're reading my book, so I'm just going to assume that I like you. So what if you meet someone who doesn't? Fuck 'em, they've got bad taste.

2. Only chat to people who make you feel good, and ignore people who don't.

   Comedian Margaret Cho said, 'They call me Imodium, because I block assholes.' Be like Margaret Cho.

3. Don't move too fast.

   Don't be pressured into giving out your number, or into meeting before you're ready.

4. But don't move too slowly either.

   So, you're getting along? Arrange to meet as soon as it's convenient for you. The more you chat, the higher your expectations, and the greater the disappointment if they turn out not to be right for you. Don't leave it so long that it gets awkward.

5. Tactical ghosting.

   If you haven't even met yet, the chats are boring, you haven't exchanged numbers or you're not feeling it, I don't think you need to explain yourself. Quietly unmatch and move on.

6. Have an adventure.

    A date is the perfect opportunity to go somewhere you've never been and try something you've always wanted to, whether it's that vegan tapas place that's just opened or a day out at the Cheddar Gorge Cheese Company. (This is a genuine first date recommendation from a friend of mine.)

How to reject someone nicely

Apparently, Socrates came up with 'the test of three': before you open your mouth, ask yourself – is what I'm about to say kind, necessary and true? If it doesn't meet at least two of those criteria, don't say it. Pretty good rule of thumb, if you ask me.

It's important to be honest when we feel that we don't want to pursue a relationship with someone, but how do we do it?

A few years ago, after going on a few dates with a very nice man, I received the following text:

I've just been asked by another date if we can be exclusive, and I'd like to see where it goes, so I'm really sorry but I'm going to have to stop seeing you. I had a lot of fun, thank you lovely and good luck xx

Naturally, I was a little disappointed. He had a killer smile and a lovely little bum like two eggs in a hanky, and I was hoping I'd get to know him better. But what a marvellous way to be let down. There was no fey talk of 'slowing things down'; he wasn't 'really busy at work', nor was he 'confused' about what he wanted. He conveyed the truth, directly and kindly. What more can anyone ask? Empathetic honesty doesn't mean being evasive. It doesn't mean being selective with the truth. You can communicate sensitive information while treating the recipient with dignity and compassion.

How an emotionally abusive relationship affected my mental health

When I was 18, I was approached by a boy in a nightclub. He was five years older than me, handsome, worldly and very confident. He became my first boyfriend and I was with him for three years. I thought it meant he loved me when he chipped away at me little by little, sneering at my love of theatre, comparing being an actress to being a prostitute, buying me new clothes to replace the ones he didn't like, withholding physical affection and underplaying our relationship (he never referred to me as his girlfriend), while wanting to know where I was and who I was with every minute of the day and night. I thought it meant he loved me when he accused me of sleeping with everyone we knew – including, when I didn't answer my phone for an hour, my driving instructor. I had my own place, but he always insisted that we spend our time on his turf, which stank of cat shit and weed and where we'd sit in, night after night. He still lived with his mum, so we were rarely alone. I gradually stopped seeing my friends, and saw less and less of my own family.

I thought all this meant that he truly loved me. I soon became utterly infatuated with him, being very young and very silly. I just didn't know any better.

It wasn't until I went to uni at 21 that I got some eye-opening perspective on this relationship. I realised how far away from myself I'd willingly been led. My new friends' boyfriends made the effort to come and visit them, rather than insisting on home visits every weekend. They didn't sulk at their girlfriends for going on a night out. They didn't bully them or threaten to dump them, or belittle them in front of their own friends.

During the first Christmas break, I was at my sister's house. She was nine months pregnant, and my two-year-old niece followed her around the kitchen imitating her wide-legged waddle and demanding the attention that she seemed to intuit would soon be divided in half. I was trying to keep her occupied when my boyfriend called. When I told him I was busy looking after my niece, he screamed at me for not paying attention to him and slammed the phone down.

My heart dropped like a stone. I knew I had been so unhappy for such a long time, but this felt like a new kind of… *wrong*. When I told my Mam how I was feeling she gently asked 'Do you think you'd like to break up with him?' And I was shocked at the notion. It honestly hadn't occurred to me before that I had a choice in the matter. That I could leave.

I ended our relationship a few days later, on New Year's Eve, five days before my second niece was born. To my surprise, he cried. After I left him, he called and called until I turned off my phone. He turned up at my parents' door the next day. Over the next few weeks he sent daily emails and letters. He changed his tone with each one – one day he'd be pleading, the next he'd be romantic or cajoling or stern. He promised me the world – holidays in far-flung locations, or our own place together. I was going to see a whole new him, he claimed. Shortly after that he sent me pictures of himself with two extremely bored-looking strippers ('They're mother and daughter! THROWING themselves at me!').

I didn't engage with him, because I couldn't. I was exhausted from giving him so much of myself over three years. I had nothing left to give. Eventually he left me alone. To this day I make a point of celebrating New Year's Eve. I'll never forget that night on the bus home from Wrexham, crying to my mam, who told me, 'Come home, love. I've made you a nice tea, and there's a bottle of Cava in the fridge.'

That formative experience has shaped the person I am now. At 21 I promised myself that I'd never put a man's needs over my own ever again. And I never have. It instilled in me the need to catch up, a fierce sense that I have to suck the marrow out of everything life has to offer. It's made me brave. Nothing grinds you down like powerlessness in a relationship, a job, even a particularly unpleasant house-share. If you feel helpless, please reach out to someone you trust. With the right support, you can take steps to reclaim your power and prioritise your own mental wellness.

That Tinder date that went viral

A decade later, I went on a first – and only – date with a man I met on Tinder. The next day he said some pretty horrible things about my weight ('my mind gets turned on by someone slimmer... I'd marry you like a shot if you were a slip of a girl'). I suspect he might regret that now because I wrote a blog about it, which went on to get over 500,000 views. My Instagram feed skyrocketed from 70 to 30,000 followers in a week. I was in the national and global press, from Australia to New York, and while I was sent countless messages of support and solidarity, the trolls got busy too. Loads of people accused me of lying (because, you know, women always do, don't they?). The one thing that really affected me was being trashed in a national newspaper in the UK for having criticised my Tinder date for rejecting me because of my size. The point is, I didn't. What I objected to was him sending me a text, after one date, explaining in forensic detail that he didn't find me sexually attractive because of my figure (I'm a size 14–16, the size of the average woman in the UK). His message was not just about his physical preference, or to tell me there wouldn't be a second date. It was an assertion of power. The subtext was, 'I could love you thiiiiiiiiiiiis much... if only you were different.' It's a strategy used by some individuals (and even some corporations) to corrode the self-esteem of others until they feel powerless. And this strategy will continue to be very effective until we stop being ashamed of our bodies because we're too fat, too thin, too short, too scarred, or too different.

This experience, and the insane pressure of the world's response to my story, could have had a terrible impact on my mental health. I've received thousands of messages from people all over the world who felt that they might never recover from similar incidents of bullying. I will always be proud that my little blog flew around the world and into the hearts of many, and in so doing, triggered a media conversation about unacceptable dating behaviour.

How to love a mad person V.1

When I fell seriously mentally ill while at the comedy company, the man who loved me at the time was my compass. He helped me manage my madness, even though neither of us realised that that was what was happening.

Our relationship changed from being gently mutually dependent, in a 'you do the washing, I'll do the drying' way, to a far more co-dependent, unhealthy 'when are you coming home? I've got a weird rash and I need you to tell me it's not meningitis' way.

My anxiety disorder manifested itself in worrying about him. Was he eating properly? Did he get to work safely? What if he got mugged on the way home? During that time, he sent me frequent texts to reassure me that he was all right.

My mood swings were so severe they gave me mental whiplash. Every few months, I'd feel the urge to jettison everything in my life that meant the most to me. Like when you're trying to save space on your hard drive, so you delete all your pictures because they're taking up the most space.

In my head, I travelled continents every day. It was exhausting for me, so I can't imagine what it was like for him. Lonely, I guess. There was a tremendous amount of pressure on him. He didn't, or couldn't, talk to anyone about it, out of loyalty to me. He had to take care of me and of himself, all on his own. I think that my depression made me difficult to love. But he still loved me, patiently and kindly, when I needed it the most and felt I deserved it the least. And I'll always be grateful to him for that.

How to love a mad person V.2

After I broke up with this (brilliant and kind) partner of six years, I needed somewhere to put all the love I still felt. I needed someone to worry about, to give my anxiety something to do and stop it from eating me alive. So, I decided to love a friend of mine who was also mad. He'd tried to die, you see, and I wanted to help him want to be alive again. It was *so* unhealthy, but it worked for a little while because we were both extremely sad at the same time. And we knew it was finite – he was on the road to recovery and was moving to a different city.

We're still friends. He's far away, but he's still one of my favourite people. I will always think he's marvellous. We both agree that our relationship was 'the best unhealthy thing we've ever done'.

Single, and please don't make me mingle

Emma Morano, who before her death at the age of 117 was the world's oldest living person, credited her long life to over 70 years of singledom.

After the end of her marriage in 1938, Emma had a few suitors but never settled down again. To a habitual dater and serial monogamist like myself, this feat of independence seems positively other-worldly. How did she spend all that time? What did she talk to her coupled-up friends about? I'm sorry, but you can only feign an interest in other people's children for so long.

I decided to try and stay single for one year (a 'dick detox', as one friend charmingly put it). I learned that while I can, of course, get by perfectly well on my own, life gets a bit boring without a special someone to send memes to.

For the first three months, I was a living Bodyform advert. I ran a half marathon. I started talking therapy. I created a

WhatsApp group called 'Gym Bitches' where we, to this day, bully each other into attending spin classes. I felt healthier and happier than I had in years.

Then two things happened. First, I developed a horrible, all-consuming crush on a pop star whose music I don't even like. I was so genuinely concerned about the strength of my feelings that I told my therapist about them, half-suspecting that she might have to break her code of confidentiality and put me on some kind of police watch list for pre-offending stalkers. She reassured me that I'd cut off an extremely powerful part of myself, and this is how it was making itself known – a textbook teenage crush on an inaccessible celebrity.

But I was troubled. The power of this terrible fantasy had shaken my faith in my Strong Independent Womanhood. In another few months, my obsession could be out of control. I could end up like those sad women with poorly-drawn portraits of Westlife tattooed on their backs.

Second, I had my hair cut. The hairdresser was a tall, stylish Polish boy with the most beautiful hands. I hadn't been touched beyond a quick hug in six months. Now here was this prince, tugging my hair, dragging his gorgeous fingers over my cheeks and neck. He teased the tiny curls out from around my ears. He *actually blew* stray hairs off the back of my neck. It took every scrap of strength not to lean my face into his hands and purr. When I left the salon, cheeks aflush, my upbeat mood quickly plummeted. I was so single that a bloody *haircut* had felt obscenely intimate. And now it was over, I felt desperately lonely.

So, what happened next? I downloaded the dating apps again, matched with the gorgeous creature I mentioned at the beginning of this chapter, a handsome chap who lived nearby, and BOOM. That was it. Stupid, predictable love. Had I met the one? Of course not. After I'd stopped misinterpreting a quickening heart and oodles of adrenaline for danger and/or passion, it was over as quickly as it had started, another short and miserable relationship. Except this time, the heartbreak was laced with an added layer of humiliation. I felt I'd broken my vow for a fool, and in doing so had made a fool of myself.

I've been conditioned by society to assume that being in a relationship is something I should covet and that will massively improve my life, and it's hard to accept that, so far, that hasn't been the case. I'm very impatient. I've never mastered a musical instrument because I've never wanted to *learn* how to play one – I just want to be a rock star without doing the graft. Likewise, I don't want to have to date. I don't want to have to spend time getting to know someone if they're going to have the audacity not to be *the one*. I've got enough friends, I just want to find a husband now and tick it off my list of things to do. It's terribly unromantic, I know. But what can I say? I'm a busy woman.

A word on terrible men

'I'm not looking for a relationship right now. I just want to hang around with someone and have fun, y'know?'

'I just want someone to invest a lot of, like, time and effort in making me feel good, but I don't want to have to give anything back.'

'Sure, I wanna check in with someone every day.

Share the little things. That, to me, is an important part of the single experience. No pressure, no labels.'

Throw them to the sharks and keep on fishing, I say.

* * *

So how does your mental health affect your relationships?

Ashley
It is definitely a struggle parenting with mental illness

My husband and I got counselling to work through our issues – my terrible self-image, his residual insecurities from past relationships. After ten years together I've just been diagnosed with bipolar II and anxiety. My husband's therapist suggested that he is co-dependent. Fortunately for us we work very hard at creating our own style of parenting and at maintaining our relationship, striving for a healthier dynamic and doing our best to heal ourselves and end the dysfunction in our families with our generation.

My girls are five and eight. It is definitely a struggle parenting with mental illness. Sometimes you really need time alone, and you simply cannot get it. I want to be free from distraction to manage my anxiety, and I find it tremendously difficult to be a person who is pleasant to be around when I'm doing this. One way I handle this is to use sound-cancelling headphones.

We haven't expressly spoken with the kids about our mental illness issues – they're a bit young. We don't hide anything from them, though. They hear us saying, 'OK, my anxiety is flaring. I need to go and take a minute alone,' and they see us employing breathing techniques and mantras and the like. My youngest also has anxiety, so she has done therapy and has been taught some coping skills as well, and we try to do them together when she's acting out. What we are learning together as a family is how to change some of the practices my husband and I learned from our families. This effort is really an attempt to ensure that our children, and we ourselves for that matter, feel heard, accepted and loved.

Megan
I tried to keep my OCD a secret whenever I got into a relationship

My OCD [obsessive compulsive disorder] was triggered when I was 13, and I suffered from it on and off for a little over ten years before I finally got proper help. Without getting too explicit, my OCD involves intrusive sexual thoughts. For years, I tried to keep it a secret whenever I got into a relationship, mostly out of fear that my partner wouldn't understand what I was going through and would leave me. When I finally got the help I needed, I started to feel more comfortable talking about it and decided that I wanted to be more open about it.

The results have been kind of a mixed bag. There was a time I told a guy I was casually seeing that I had OCD, and he responded with, 'Oh, me too! I'm such a neat freak and have to have everything in a certain order. I'm so OCD.' It crushed me a bit to hear this, and I spent the next few minutes trying to explain to him that that's not how OCD really works, and why it was offensive to say that. We didn't date for long after that.

Towards the end of a different relationship, my OCD got so bad that I wasn't leaving my apartment for days on end. Every conversation I had with my boyfriend at the time became difficult, because we were both trying to avoid the subject and also trying to talk it out. It was brutal on us both.

On the flip side, I've also been lucky to have really supportive responses from romantic partners. One of my past boyfriends suffered from depression and anxiety, so while he didn't always understand how my OCD worked, he definitely related to my struggles and tried to help me when I needed it. Another guy I dated didn't always understand, but he constantly made the effort to listen to me and to absorb everything I said. These moments made me feel so understood and loved, and I think they're one of the reasons I'm able to tell my story today.

Gregg

Hypersexuality is part of depression sometimes

One thing that didn't fade out during my depression was my libido. Which isn't good, because if you're really not doing well physically or mentally there's no chance you can talk to or hook up with anyone in a healthy way. So I got into having one-night stands, which I look back on now as out of character for me. At the time, because of the frame of mind I was in, I'd alienated my family and my friends, I couldn't work, I felt like shit and nothing made sense. So, because nothing made any sense, I started making decisions that didn't make any sense to match – 'I'm probably dying and everything sucks, so I might as well take MDMA every day for a week.' I got into some unwise sexual situations during that time, with some sketchy people. I'd hang out in this drugs-and-sex house where people just, like, go and hang out and do drugs and have sex, just an ongoing grim depressing house party that didn't end. So, I'd go there and take a bunch of drugs and have loads of sex with randomers. But hypersexuality is part of depression sometimes.

Mariel
My husband has taught me that sadness is something you can struggle with forever while also having a pretty good life

I grew up in a family that doesn't name depression or anxiety and is more likely to say, 'Suck it up' than, 'You should go see someone about this.'

My husband suffers from pretty severe depression and anxiety. He got so bad at one point that he couldn't even tie his shoes. He bent down to do it after I had talked him into taking a walk, and he just cried and cried. He wasn't himself.

My husband has taught me that sadness is something you can struggle with forever while also having a pretty good life.

We don't talk about it during good times, because we don't need to. We have had countless conversations about it when he is suffering. I think the most important thing to remember is that when it happens, it affects his perception. He feels hopeless for a minute or an hour, but then he knows he will be OK. I just watch. Sometimes I call his parents to talk to him. That helps. Once I called the doctor and got him in. That was a big help, too. Once I wrote a letter to him instead of talking.

He takes maybe six different pills a day – for depression, anxiety, ADD [attention deficit disorder], high blood pressure.

He has side effects and the pills don't always work. And he fears that he is not his real self when medicated. I say he is. I think the medication pushes back the scary things in his brain, so his real self can come out. I love meds because I love my husband. Even when he is very dark or sad, he always has moments when anyone would love him.

My husband was diagnosed with emotionally unstable personality disorder, PTSD and anxiety a year after we got together. At first, the impact on our relationship was huge. He didn't want to talk. He made multiple attempts at suicide and smashed the house up in psychosis. We were both drained and felt alone. We couldn't enjoy a normal relationship because he was so unwell and I was so exhausted and scared for him. Once he opened up, things got lots better. We became closer and our relationship of nine years is now strong and built on deep trust and the ability to support one another. He takes quetiapine, which literally knocks him out – we can no longer have late-night walks or film binges, and we have to schedule our sex life around his meds. But in return I have an incredible, funny, happy, healthy and stable husband, so it's a small price to pay. Learning about Tom's mental health has inspired me, given me a whole new understanding of what love and marriage mean, and has made me really appreciate the good days. I think we have a deeper level of love and understanding than either of us have ever had in relationships without mental illness. We argue less, because we've had to learn great communication to help manage his anxiety and his emotional rawness. We're now planning a family and I believe his experiences with mental illness will make him the kindest, most caring and compassionate father anyone could wish for.

My Shit Body

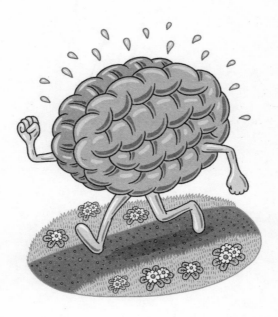

I SPRAINED MY ANKLE A COUPLE OF YEARS AGO. I PHONED the hospital, and was advised to go to A&E. I texted my boss at the pub and explained my injury (throwing in a pic of my grotesquely swollen ankle for good measure). He wished me a speedy recovery and found cover for the next few shifts, so that I could rest and recuperate. At A&E, I was assessed by a triage nurse, who arranged for me to have an X-ray. I was then sent to see a physiotherapist, who carefully examined my ankle, advised me to buy some high-top trainers to support it, and told me to keep off my feet for at least three days and not to run for at least two to three weeks. When I was ready to re-engage with my day-to-day life, allowances were made to make it easier for me to physically navigate the world in new circumstances. Friends and family asked what had happened, how I was feeling, how they could help. If I'd had a cast, people would have signed it. Visible illness and visible trauma are recognisable and undeniable.

Imagine if the same allowances were made for mental and emotional trauma. Imagine guilt-free time to rest and let your mind recuperate. Imagine seeing your GP for a same-day assessment, diagnosis and advice before you reach crisis point, without facing a potentially long wait to talk to an expert. Imagine having the resources available to fix yourself. Imagine asking for help with no fear of stigma, judgement or shame. It would be so much easier to manage your madness before it escalated. Mental health days off in addition to your annual leave allocation would be a start.

Body issues

According to the NHS, one in four of us in the UK is overweight. I am one of the one in four, but I don't really mind. Everything's in the right place, and everything works. I'd like to get a bit fitter, but that's not to say that I don't love and enjoy my body right now. Here. Today.

Your body should never, ever be a source of shame. You can decide you want to change your body for the better, but taking care of it doesn't mean you have to hurt it. It doesn't mean starving it, wearing it out, gorging that beautiful brain which you should be filling with books and art and driving lessons instead of identical, dead-eyed, alien images which imply that being tall and white and skinny and never smiling is the only way for any woman to be of any worth.

Absolutely no good comes from hating your body. You must train yourself to love it. It is not an object, nor a commodity; neither is it a burden. It is not someone else's trophy. It's the only thing in this world that is uniquely yours, and you only get one. Sadly, there are people – rich, powerful people – who aim to make a lot of money from tricking you into thinking of your body as a source of shame. They will tell you that it's too big, too hairy, too pale, too dark, too muscly, or not muscly enough. There are individuals who will try to use this awful power to undermine you, to control and manipulate you. Do not let them. Challenge them. Outwit them. Show them your disdain for them. But above all, laugh at them. Then you'll have won. We will ALL have won.

Two ways to beat the body-shamers

Fix your feed

The beauty of social media is that you can curate your own experience. Rather than buying a glossy fashion magazine and flicking through 200 pages of similar images, you can tailor your feed to show you the world as you want to see it, and marvel at all the infinitely diverse ways people can be happy, healthy, smart, witty, kind and beautiful. With Instagram, you can find out how people live in the remotest corners of the earth. You can follow the Guggenheim, the Tate, the V&A, and see world-class art every single day, wherever you are, for free. No generation has had that privilege before. It's easy to sneer that Insta is all cats, brunch, selfies and beach yoga, but social media is one of the most powerful tools for self-education we have.

If your feed is boring you, don't blame the tool or the algorithms. If you're choosing to be spoon-fed, you can't complain that everything tastes the same.

Instagram has a reputation for exacerbating poor body image, but it's honestly my favourite place to hang out online.

Who I follow on Instagram

Powerful women

Polly Nor, illustrator (pollynor)
She says she 'draws women and their demons' and I've never seen a more accurate bio. Her artwork is stunning.

She recently created a 39-post epic thriller, eking it out with one post per day over six weeks.

Stina Wollter, performance artist (stinawollter)
She dances in her underwear and with her mum.

The Mirnavator (themirnavator)
Growing up, I didn't see any women with a body like mine who were physically fit, sporty, deft, and graceful. Mirna Valerio is a 200-pound woman who runs ultra-marathons. And every time I see her doing stuff I didn't think women who looked like me could do, I feel my brain creating a new neuropathway with a truthful view of what 'healthy' looks like.

Eye feasts

Miranda Tacchia (mrmtacchia)
Rude, raunchy, hilarious comics.

Zen Pencils (zenpencils)
Exquisitely executed comics, based on words of wisdom from history's greatest minds. Check out Sylvia Plath and Ballet Boy.

Good eggs

Jack Monroe (bootstrapcook_)
ALL THE FOODSTUFFS!

Hemmo (hemmograms)
Her book *Running Like a Girl* inspired me to finish the Couch to 5k, then go on to 10k, then a half marathon.

She also writes about swimming in the sea like an absolute badass.

Technically Ron (technicallyron)
You can follow him on Twitter, too. His book about mental health is in the sources section. It's awfully good.

Silver Pebble (silverpebble2)
Author, naturalist and illustrator. Very soothing, very beautiful and very British.

Funnies

Yes, I'm Hot in This (yesimhotinthis)
Webcomic about the musings of Huda F, 'a slightly sweaty Muslim-American woman'.

Alec with Pen (alecwithpen)
Weird. Wild. Very funny.

Awards for Good Boys (awardsforgoodboys)
Such delicious snark.

Things that have absolutely nothing to do with mental health

Color Palette Cinema (colorpalette.cinema)
Literal colour palettes that match some of the most beautiful shots in cinema.

Trejo's Coffee & Donuts (trejosdonuts)
Danny Trejo (of *Machete* fame) and doughnuts. What's not to love?

Focus on what your body can do, not what it looks like

Start a Couch to 5k workout regime. Try Zumba. Do a free 30-day yoga challenge on YouTube. Look into zorbing, or live-action role-playing, or discorobics. It doesn't matter how you use your body, just enjoy all the amazing things you can do with it.

How have body issues affected your mental health?

Nutritionist Sophie Pelham Burn told me, 'I hear an awful lot about body image and shape every day. A lot of what I hear is people being negative about their own bodies, driven by what they hear in the media... I also hear people berating others for "not taking care of themselves". Often those comments are well-meaning, but that doesn't make them any less destructive, or factually incorrect! With the use of hashtags across social media, we're seeing more and more "fitspo"-[health blogs and images] type influences on top of the pre-existing high fashion pressures that have been prevalent for decades. These additional influences assume body weight to be a proxy indicator for health, which is simply not true. Skinny does not equal healthy, and neither does athleticism.'

I've received too many messages from women and men battling everything from anorexia and bulimia to addiction and over-exercising, and from others who are so paralysed by shame and depression from being overweight or obese that they don't know what to do other than hide themselves away and eat, and eat, and eat, and eat. In both extremes, these people discuss learning this behaviour from parents, older siblings, boyfriends, girlfriends or best friends. Each cites an occasion where they were bullied and shamed for the way their body looked – at the ages of seven, nine, 13 – long before their illness took hold. I've also received too many messages from 12-year-old girls, expressing displeasure, disgust and concern about what their bodies look like now, and what they may look like in the future. They're terrified of gaining weight. They're not terrified of getting cancer or losing a loved one. The worst thing – the very worst thing – they can imagine is getting fat. Or rather, other people thinking they're fat.

My body: a chronology

1993

I'm a ponderous, cautious, serious kid who doesn't mix well with others my age. I live entirely in my own brain, in books, in stories. I've no interest in the kinetic world – in fact, I'd like to move as little as possible. I really want one of those reclining beds for old people that I've seen in adverts. I quite like the idea of being an invalid. Having a body seems like a very tedious bit of life admin. I discover that I'm fat when I'm nine years old. I am informed of this fact by a girl in my year at primary school:

'Michelle, I'd be lying if I said you weren't fat,'

I feel sick.

'I know,' I reply in a whisper.

Actually, I hadn't known I was fat until she told me, but I didn't want her to know that.

It's so unfair. I don't like having a body. It seems to me that other people don't like my having a body either. So I begin to pretend I simply don't have one. I ignore it, try to disappear into the background as best I can, and keep my head down and buried in a book.

1997

I'm 12, and I'm fascinated by *Titanic* star Kate Winslet. She's extremely pretty and she has bosoms and a belly and a bum. She looks like some of the girls in sixth form, the girls I want to look like when I grow up.

Those pictures of then-22-year-old Winslet in a strappy, lacy, curve-hugging dress at the *Titanic* premiere are in the national papers for weeks. Gradually, I start to pay attention to what is being written about my new hero (I hadn't actually seen the film by this point. I just knew she must be a star because of all the attention she was getting for the way she looked). I read the way her body is judged and scrutinised in tones that swing between common sense ('She looks like a woman! A normal, healthy, human woman!') and deep distrust (I read rumours of certain (male) actors and directors refusing to work with her unless she loses weight).

One article debates Kate's premiere dress – 'Was It Hot or Not?' This is the first time I have interpreted 'curves' as a negative. Kate Winslet seems to be on the receiving end of a grown-up version of the taunts I receive at school. I remember looking at the pictures of her after reading those critical words, at 12 years old, and thinking, 'Actually… maybe they're right. She *shouldn't* have worn that. She *is* a bit too voluptuous [another word I learn that week]. She's really pretty, but if she lost weight, then she'd be perfect. She'd look like a real star.' My child's mind is weighing and measuring Kate Winslet with the assistance of the media's endless comparisons to her thinner contemporaries. And I remember thinking, 'If *she's* fat, what hope do I have?'

1998

I fear and abhor physical exercise. I feel like a different species from every other girl in my year, especially the sporty girls. Given that we're in rural Wales, there are also many girls who live on farms. Girls who can carry hay bales and fence posts. Girls who spend their weekends traversing acres of land to mend fences and tend to the livestock. Strong, seemingly unselfconscious girls who seem to understand that their bodies are tools. Machines. Equipment.

I dodge PE classes at school every Monday and Thursday for about two months because I feel I simply cannot do it. It doesn't feel like a lie when I tell my parents I'm ill – the anxiety is genuinely nauseating. The tears are real.

In hindsight, of course I could have done PE. My body was normal for a girl my age, but I didn't like the way it looked when it moved. I didn't like the way it looked when it was still, either. Really, I was still pretending I didn't have a body. It was easier than examining how I really felt about it. And it wasn't the thought of engaging in physical exercise that terrified me. It was the thought of being watched and judged during PE, and found lacking. It didn't occur to me that everyone in the class would be too busy to watch and judge me. In my anxious and utterly self-obsessed teenage mind, I'd convinced myself that I would be a target. At least when I managed to dodge PE, I'd sit at home and read and read until my brain was as full as an egg.

2004

I am through to the final round of auditions for a prestigious drama school. The audition is before a Shakespeare scholar – a man who knows every letter of every word Shakespeare ever wrote (and quite a few that he may not have). I've chosen Cleopatra for my monologue because she is a Strong Woman (I have recently become an enthusiastic advocate of Strong Women). I sit and watch Mr Scholar tear strips off participants who stand and speak beautifully, but aren't really engaged in the meaning of the words. (It sounds obvious, but an actor really should understand the meaning of their lines. I once auditioned for a Welsh-language Shakespeare play where a terribly pretty, terribly dim boy recited the line, 'You kissed me once, on the lips' and pointed at his forehead.)

I am brimming with anxiety, but I can't wait to perform for this man. There aren't many things I'm confident that I'm good at, but my aptitude for book-learning means that I probably know my shit better than anyone else in this room. I know THEIR speeches better than they do, and I know I can withstand any interrogation about any editorial revisions. I am nothing if not formidably nerdy. I also know Cleopatra, the famous Egyptian leader, as best a 19-year-old Welsh lass can. I know her pride. I know her churlishness. I know her sorrow. (I'm not saying I'm the lost Judi Dench of my generation. Although I could be. We'll never know. I'm just saying I worked hard.)

I begin my audition. I keep my voice steady, my tone rich. I move around the space as I've been directed to by my drama teacher ('using the space' is very important in The Theatre), drawing imaginary pentagrams with my feet, keeping my mind's eye on the faithless Anthony, goading him, taunting him.

'Eternity was in our lips and eyes,
Bliss in our brows' bent, none our parts so poor
But was a race of heaven...'

'NO. NO. NO. YOU'RE MAKING YOUR BODY LOOK UGLY,' he booms around the auditorium.

My breath stops as I turn to stare at the great scholar. His words are suspended in the air like icicles. No one else seems to think he's said anything outrageous or unacceptable, so maybe he's right. It takes me a fraction of a second to snap out of my shock, to recompose my body language, to ask cheerily, 'OK! What can I do to change that?' I don't remember exactly how he responds, just a stream of stage directions that I don't take in. What I can still remember is the horror – the dry, inevitable horror – of having my fears confirmed. I am pretending to be the woman frequently idealised as the most beautiful who ever lived, and I'm failing because I can't even *pretend* to be the right kind of beautiful. So it doesn't matter how well I know the play, how hard I've worked, it doesn't matter that I've lived with those stories in my heart and those words in my mouth for months. I'm not able to do what I yearn for, because I don't even know how to pretend to make my body look beautiful.

2013

I start running after I experience my first major depressive episode. I start running because I'm terrified, and I need a practical strategy to fix my brain. Leaving the flat feels like agony. I run for 60 seconds at a time, praying for respite between intervals of walking along sad grey pavements. There are no endorphins, just numb relief when I'm finally allowed to go home and cry in the bath.

2015

I can run for an hour and a half without stopping or dying, and I'm bloody delighted. It's taken two belligerent, bloody-minded years for me to stop thinking of running as a chore; for the chorus of 'This-is-bullshit-this-is-bullshit-this-is-BULLshit' to stop chugging through my head as I wheeze and pant around the neglected South London park. I'd run regularly for a few weeks at a time, then stop because it was too hard or I was too lazy. I never put my trainers on without seething resentment weighing me down. But a lot has changed in the two years since my meltdown. I've left a promising-but-unfulfilling career as an agent to make lattes in a cafe and write. My long-term relationship has ended. I've been on holiday on my own. I've lost 15lb. Now I put my headphones on when I go out running, and it's just me and my legs and my lungs and the road and the sky.

* * *

I still grapple with the notion that I have to be good at running, that it's not enough to just *do* it. When I'm running I often notice toddlers in the park, roaring and rampaging and chasing squirrels and running with no destination and no impetus beyond, 'Look there's a leaf I must dance with it and what happens if I stretch my hands up in the air and go BLAAAAARGH! This is fantastic I'm going to keep doing it BLAAAAAAARGH!!!' It's play. It's instinct. They are learning how to be human, and part of that means grasping the mechanics of their bodies, the vessel they're in. I must have done that once. But when you've spent so many years avoiding exercise because you're terrible at it, it takes an enormous psychological shift to overcome that fear. I avoided it for so long, because moving my body meant admitting that I'd had one all along, and that I'd been neglecting it. It's like checking your bank balance at the end of a decadent month; but when you haven't checked your body for 30 years, it's your life expectancy that you might discover is much lower than you thought.

My first 10k

According to the amazing This Girl Can campaign, run by Sport England, the fear of judgement from others is the primary barrier holding women back from participating in sport. This fear concerns their appearance, ability, or being seen to choose to spend time on themselves, rather than on their families. Sport England's research reveals that from an early age, appearance is a concern for women when it comes to exercise. Thirty-six per cent of the least-active school girls that their body is on show in PE lessons, and that makes them like PE less. One woman in every four says 'I hate the way I look when I exercise' or play sport.

How utterly sad that women and girls are less likely to enjoy the mental and physical benefits of regular exercise, partly because they fear being judged for the way they look. Our bodies are an integral part of our life experience. They're the connective tissue between our brains and our souls and all the wonderful things we have to enjoy in this world. So my attitude is, if you feed your brain and soul but neglect your body, you'll only ever live two-thirds of your life.

I signed up to my first 10k eight weeks in advance, when I'd just hit 5k and wanted a new challenge. Over two months I trained three times a week, adding five minutes per week. My body felt like a new toy. I remember the triumph of running for 30 minutes, then 40, then 55. I was thrilled that I could run for a whole 25 minutes as a compromise on the odd days when I really couldn't be bothered, when a short time earlier it had taken every fraction of my stamina to reach that. I was slow, but so what? My first 5k took 40 mins, so I aimed to do 10k in 90 minutes. I didn't really care how long it took; I didn't care if I came last. I wanted to run the whole 10k, no stops, no walks.

The run wasn't particularly well organised, and neither was I. It wasn't until the day before that I realised I had no information about start times or meeting places. When I searched online I discovered that there would be no trains running early enough for the 8am start time, so I had to arrange for an expensive cab to pick me up at 6.30am to allow for time to queue up for the racing number I still didn't have. But that wasn't the only nasty discovery I made.

'This race has a maximum time of 1hr 15 mins.'

This was because the lanes needed to be clear for the half-marathon runners who had a later start time. Also... race? I'd signed up for a run – an act of running for a set distance, nothing more. Now it was a race – a running *competition* – with a time limit I was certain I couldn't meet. I packed and repacked my bag – plasters, water, raincoat, hairpins, Rescue Remedy – certain I'd forget something important, I wouldn't be allowed to run, and I'd let down my charity (Mind, of course) and all the people who'd sponsored me.

On race day, I felt sick with nerves. I was tense and irritable. I didn't want to be around anyone, particularly not 300 racers, each one looking as though they knew exactly what they were doing, swigging coconut water and doing special sexy stretches in special sexy pants with mesh panels behind the knee for strategic breathability. One runner was wearing knickers – actual running knickers, like British running champion Paula Radcliffe. *They must chafe like a bastard after the 40-minute mark*, I thought wanly. After an inaudible announcement that I took to mean, 'The race is about to start,' we shuffled to the start line. Although I'd studied the map, I'd already lost what little sense of direction I had. I had no idea which way I was running, so I asked the women in front of me.

'Just follow the crowd!' they beamed at me.

Their kind smiles thawed the knot in my diaphragm, and I realised I was excited. I'd noticed one of the women earlier. She was a strikingly large woman, her size-24 frame enrobed in fluorescent yellow Lycra.

'Are you running for a charity?' I asked her.

'No, it's a personal challenge,' she grinned.

Adele was running 1,000km – 600 miles – in the year between her 39th and 40th birthday. She was halfway through, running a combination of 10k and half-marathons. I told them it was my first 10k.

'It's a great achievement. It's a very emotional thing, too – don't be surprised if you cry at the end. Good luck. Enjoy it!'

The race began, and my queue friends ran off ahead of me. As did the 300 other participants. I'm slow, I always knew I'd be slow, and I always said it didn't matter if I came last as long as I finished, but I've never been more daunted than I felt then, left behind in the dust. There was one man running behind me as I trotted along the almost-empty course. When I came to a crossroads, I stopped. There was no signposting.

'Straight ahead!' the man behind me called. 'Over the bridge, then follow the other stewards!'

I turned around and looked at him. My running mate was a steward, making sure the runtiest wildebeest in the herd found her way to the watering hole. I thanked him and jogged on, alone. Already there were uber-runners speeding back for their second lap, their legs working like pistons. I felt a little envious, but more than that, I was fascinated to watch ordinary people running. What they wore. How they moved their arms. Whether they managed the perfect mid-foot strike (I run on my heels – an awful habit, I'm told). All ages, all body shapes. And yes, I may have been the weediest runner in the pack, but at that moment I was so proud to be part of it that I honestly didn't care.

The race was split into two 5k laps. It took me 40 minutes to finish the first, by which time I really was on my own. With no signposts and no stewards on hand, I found myself back at the start line, where the half-marathoners were gathering, snorting out hot steam and pawing the ground in ergonomic high-end trainers. I was lost, and alarmed. If the half-marathon started now I'd be swept up in the stampede. I'd die, like Mufasa in *The Lion King*. Anxiety welled up in me again. I couldn't find my track, I couldn't find a steward, and was losing time – I needed to finish. In desperation, I elbowed my way down a side street and nipped back on to the track. It may have been a tiny shortcut, but I was on the go again, and I was completely over my anxious thoughts about the other runners, what they were doing and what they thought of me. By the time the half-marathoners started overtaking me I was totally lost in my own experience. I saw Adele towards the end of her second lap and waved furiously, and nodded my appreciation at the stewards who yelled, 'Keep going!' at the last remaining 10ker. I made room for faster runners, but I didn't stop or slow down (not that I could slow down much without stopping altogether). On the final 50 metres I knew I'd done it, and a different type of wobbly anxiety filled my belly. When Adele and her friend spotted me from the finish line and started whooping in applause, I burst into tears. I held my bosom, and tried to regulate my sobs as I ran. 'Enjoy it!' yelled a steward, and I crossed the finish line to cheers. On the train home I reflected on my massive achievement. I'd run 10k! That's six miles! I'd run a mile, six times! I was still crying, but I wasn't distressed or unhappy – I cried like an ill-at-ease toddler, unable to articulate or identify my emotions. I remember that it didn't hurt, there was no physical discomfort, nor did I feel utterly exhausted. A weight had left me – I'd done it, I'd proved that I could do something that frightened me, and I clutched my medal as I hugged my knees and wept fat tears of happiness and pride.

* * *

I wanted to find out how other people's bodies had impacted their misbehaving brains, so I asked them how their mental health affected their physical health, and vice versa.

Robin
*I can't handle the things most normal people
seem to be able to*

I know I struggle with certain depression and anxiety afflictions due to my childhood, but I really feel like the bigger problem is physical. I literally feel like everything is just too much.

Like I can't handle the things most normal people seem to be able to handle, everything exhausts me. So as well as taking medication and seeing a therapist, I've also had a deep dive into my hormones and vitamins and it turns out I have a vitamin D deficiency, which can cause depression symptoms, and I may also have sleep apnea.

James
Along with the anxiety came the depression

I suffer from a debilitating physical illness, an extremely rare auto immune disease. It affects my lungs, and over the years I have had to endure a plethora of side effects such as anaemia, sepsis, blood clots and pneumonia. I coped very well on the mental health side until last year, when I had a full-on nervous breakdown after being discharged from hospital after a six-day stint of pneumonia. I had my first-ever panic attack, and I genuinely felt I was dying.

Along with the anxiety came the depression. I was ashamed of my appearance (bloated neck, chronic unfitness, body scarred from surgical knives and steroid use) and also my illness. Who would want a guy who is unable to work and provide for himself? Who has to live with his parents, because he relies on them for hospital appointments? Who is in no position to go travelling, hike up a mountain or even go for a long walk, because his lungs can't take it?

Eventually I realised that I had been neglecting my mental health, and now I am getting the support I need and making more of an effort to see friends, socialise and think realistically about my situation. I take medication for depression and anxiety, which seems to do the job. I've done some online CBT, which was OK.

Gregg

If you don't have enough glucose everything starts going wrong, and that includes your brain chemistry

I've always been kind of low-energy and gloomy. I've struggled with low moods a lot. By the time I was in my early 30s, it was really bad. At first, I thought I was just middle-aged and grumpy. My moods were fluctuating and my whole attitude to myself and the world was gradually changing because I wasn't thinking straight. I had really, really bad paranoia, I was hypervigilant, always looking around, on alert for a threat. I thought I was going mad. My short-term memory was shot. My hands would stop working – I dropped things all the time.

All these worrying symptoms put a bigger pressure on my mental health. My five-year relationship ended, because I was so paranoid and anxious all the time. I had become a different person. People invited me out and I wouldn't go, and eventually they stopped asking. I used to love meeting loads of different people. So then I moved out and lived on my own, which made it worse because I was isolated, unwell and desperate. I was incoherent, I was slurring my words, it felt like I'd lost about 100 IQ points. I was angry for no reason, I'd just wake up furious.

Eventually it got so bad that I went to my GP because it felt like I was dying. When I was in the waiting room I saw a poster about diabetes in children. And I had every single symptom. The GP agreed to do a quick blood test. A healthy blood sugar level is under 7mg. Mine was 34. They rushed me to hospital. It was really scary – I had a drip in each arm for days, while they reset all my mineral levels.

The system that controls your hormones and your energy is linked, so if you don't have enough glucose everything starts going wrong, and that includes your brain chemistry, low serotonin, mood swings, anxiety. The link between blood sugar and low mood is massive, and not really talked about a lot.

I'd alienated everyone by being a grumpy, horrible bastard, so I was in there on my own for a few days.

I asked one of the consultants, 'What does this mean? Do I have to stop drinking alcohol?' And he just said, 'Yeah, probably', and left the room. That's a massive change in my life, which no one was talking to me about or helping me with. How can I go on a date with a girl if I can't drink?

Sol

Doctors assumed I was using again

I'm a recovering addict, and I have depression. When I was pregnant I kept losing weight. My doctor told me my unborn baby would die if I didn't eat more. So I ate and ate, but couldn't put on weight. My son was only 2kg when he was born. Doctors assumed I was using again but I wasn't, I promised them I wasn't. I begged them for help. It wasn't until I had a test by a doctor who recognised the symptoms of a thyroid problem that I was diagnosed. I had a problem with my endocrine system – an overactive thyroid. With two pills a day for six months, I gained weight. A doctor had told me I was going to kill my child because I had a problem with my thyroid. If he'd done a blood test and spoken to me properly, he'd have found this out. How many women have been misdiagnosed because they weren't properly listened to?

J

You can't expect people to understand

I have a massive problem with eating, although I don't have an issue with what I look like. I've got a terrible relationship with food. I take protein shakes and stuff to work because that's an easy way to make sure I've got something in me, otherwise I just won't remember to eat. People comment on it all the time – 'Why are you eating that shit?' – and it's like, because I'll be ill otherwise. You can't expect people to understand. I just forget, or I can't be bothered. A lot of it comes down to, 'I can't be bothered.' Eating – can't be bothered. Having a shower – can't be bothered. Getting out of bed – can't be bothered. Everything feels so hard. My phone can be on the floor by my bed and it's too much effort to pick it up. Sometimes the only thing that gets me out of bed is a cigarette.

Jane

I went into the biggest downward spiral of my life

I was 23 when I had my eldest child and 27 when I had my youngest. I was 38 when I finally found a job I liked and a social circle that didn't revolve around the school timetable. I loved it.

However, not long after I started, I suffered a slipped disc and had to have surgery. When I returned to work three months later, I felt my colleagues' attitude towards me had changed. They no longer showed support and compassion, and became awkward when I had time off for physio appointments and aftercare. I was treated like a nuisance. I started stress-eating and gained a lot of weight, which didn't aid my recovery from spinal surgery. Then I was put on a sickness procedure – one more period of sickness and I was out. My neurologist told me I would need another operation. I knew that would mean more time off, so I left employment and went into the biggest downward spiral of my life, aged 43.

My friends were patient and kind but insistent that I go and see my doctor. They said I was depressed but I didn't think I had the right to be, as I had a lovely home, a wonderful husband, two great sons and no real reason to be as miserable and empty as I was. My GP put me on 20mg of citalopram and offered me counselling. I took the medication but refused the counselling, as it just felt wrong talking about myself all the time. My GP upped my dose to 30mg, 20mg in the morning and 10mg at night. I strongly believe this medication has saved my life. At one point, I lined up all my tramadol [a prescription painkiller] and wrote three letters, then went to get a bottle of vodka from the kitchen. On the way back my eldest son rang me and we started having a chat. An hour later, I ripped up the letters and put the vodka away.

It's been ten years since I started taking citalopram. I've had further spinal surgery and my mobility is limited, but I can control the pain, which is all I can ask for. I see every potential problem with a clear head and cope with it. I'm 52 now and know my limitations. Unfortunately I doubt I'll ever work again, but I'm better and that's all that matters.

8

My Shit Habits

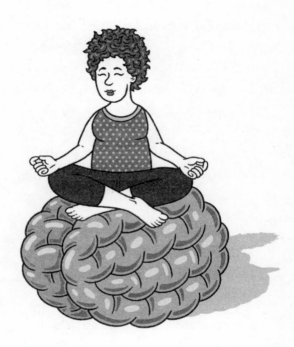

'SELF-NEGLECT IS THE ANTITHESIS OF POWER.' I HAVE NO idea who said this. Could have been Plato, could have been Dolly Parton. Either way, it's a corker of a quote to live by.

For something so wholly essential to good health and well-being, self-care is an ambiguous, catch-all, wishy-washy 'it means whatever I say it means' term. There's emptying-the-bins-and-changing-the-bedding self-care. There's green-tea-and-scented-candles self-care. There's batten-down-the-hatches-shit's-gone-down self-care. Ultimately, self-care is about humanity. It's about making decisions that protect your basic human needs – making sure you're adequately nourished, rested, exercised, and have balance between enough mental stimulation to prevent a slide into depression and not so much that you're catatonic with terror at missing a tweet. Self-care is about taking time out from your commitments to others and your work when you need it. Self-care is simple but difficult to practise, even though the consequences of self-neglect can be catastrophic for our mental health.

Depression is a rejection of the self, and this becomes the filter for every lived experience. Trying to take positive steps towards self-care when you're viewing the world through shit-tinted spectacles feels like the ultimate in futility. You don't like yourself, so you don't want to look after yourself.

During my depressive episodes in the past, I spent a lot of time bullying myself, which is about as helpful as bellowing 'STOP BEING A DICK' at your bladder when you've got a UTI. I even wrote horrible letters to myself:

This flat is filthy because of you.

You look disgusting with your massive belly and your saggy tits like a dead fucking whale.

You're so lazy you've had TWO MONTHS to write an article and you haven't bothered it's just excuses all the time it's not depression you just need to stop eating shit and exercise you can't even call your family because you're so ashamed of yourself you're not using what little talent you do have...

If anyone spoke to a friend of mine like that, I'd be at risk of spending a night in a cell. But when you're addressing yourself, and this litany is the soundtrack to every waking moment, you stop noticing. You stop caring. You don't want to buy nutritious food or wash your clothes or phone your family or empty the bin or keep your environment clean and appealing. You don't want to feel present and engaged and conscious. I'm not talking about suicidal tendencies, but when I was depressed I longed for oblivion. I just wanted to sleep, to opt out of the day. When you have depression, the act of doing anything serves as a reminder of all the things that you're not doing and being. Any act of self-care serves as a reminder that you don't care about yourself; in fact you hate yourself, because you're the worst person who ever lived. Worse than mass murderers, or even people who say 'wine o'clock'. What little energy you have is spent criticising your every action. The most banal activity is met with a barrage of self-inflicted mental abuse: *Emptying the bins, are you? What took you so long? Put yourself on the kerb while you're at it, shithead.*

I was ill, so I ignored and rejected and neglected my physical and mental health until I became even more ill.

Sound familiar? Of course it does. When we're busy or stressed – moving to a new house or caring for a new baby or dealing with a bereavement or starting a new job or ending a relationship – self-care is often the last thing we prioritise. It's quicker and easier to eat toast and margarine three times a day than it is to plan your meals, source the ingredients, lovingly cook your chosen recipe and mindfully chew every mouthful a dozen times. It feels nicer to collapse on the sofa with a bottle of wine and rip open a bag of crisps than it does to go for a run. It seems productive and valiant and boast-worthy to spend an hour catching up on emails, or to have another drink with friends you haven't seen in months, than to have an early night. Self-care means making decisions that seem to only benefit ourselves, and most of us don't want to seem selfish enough to do that, particularly in our period of late capitalism that fetishises busy-ness, idolises those who 'go the extra mile', the strivers, the hustlers, those who live on caffeine and sleep deprivation.

It's no surprise that lifestyles like the one I used to have contribute to the poor state of our collective mental health. Today great strides are being made to fight the stigma associated with mental illness, especially in the workplace. Corporations are tripping over themselves to demonstrate their credentials in tolerating and supporting a diverse workforce. When offices in London's Canary Wharf were equipped with an onsite therapy suite for stressed bankers, one of the company's board members allegedly said at its opening, 'Every morning I take an antihistamine and an antidepressant, and without either of those pills I wouldn't be able to do my job.' While anything that makes it easier to talk about mental health in the workplace is a step in the right direction, these initiatives aren't wholly altruistic. Mental health problems at work cost the UK economy £34.9 billion in 2017. Will onsite therapy suites really help those suffering with mental health issues? Or, like onsite sleeping pods and 24-hour dry-cleaners, are they a cynical strategy to increase productivity in a culture that already demands so much from its workforce?

Brands are also desperate to capitalise on the mental health movement by selling 'wellness'. Everything from seaweed-inspired leggings that allegedly pamper your skin while you sweat, to so-called 'good mood food', is aggressively marketed at women. When did you last see mood-boosting scented candles aimed at men?

A well-known organic luxury label has built a cult following, on the premise of promoting 'well-being'. The company recently released a video of the founder in conversation with a psychologist who is on their 'well-being board'. In it, the psychologist talks the viewer through the signs of stress that can affect mental health – irritability, tearfulness, reliance on alcohol (or as she casually puts it, 'an extra glass of wine in the evening'), relationship breakdown, and how these can culminate in stress-related diseases. It's asserted that nine out of ten women are affected by this kind of stress. In closing, the founder turns to camera and says, 'If this sounds like you, we can help you cope naturally,' and directs viewers to their website. One of the 'mood-boosting' products on this website is a candle, which promises to deliver a 'more positive, uplifted state of mind'. It costs £300. The company is targeting an audience who quite literally have money to burn. It's fine that there are people who want to spend a week's wages on a candle, but these gimmicks reflect an insultingly shallow approach to mental illness. I suspect these products are for people who privately believe that depression is the same as simply feeling a bit sad, and that anxiety is what happens when your selfie doesn't get enough likes. In my view, this version of wellness insinuates that anything that can't be 'cured' with a quick jog in your new leggings and a chia seed smoothie is a 'proper illness', serious and incurable, further alienating those whose mental illness requires clinical treatment.

Of course, having nice things might temporarily alleviate the symptoms of depression. But you can't put 'good mental health' on your shopping list. Spending £15 on a bag of matcha tea powder isn't practising self-care, it's just giving you a shopping buzz. And calling it self-care could lead to bigger problems than buyer's remorse.

Self-care in practice: how to fix your soul when your brain is kicking your heart in the dick

When I was ill, I desperately wanted a strategy for wellness: A+B+C = no more depression. But there's no such instant solution. So I started to devise my own.

Listen to your body. It's cleverer than you are

One positive to come out of my illness is that I know the signs that indicate an impending low patch. The early symptoms are the easiest to ignore – sleeplessness, a general loss of motivation and joy and interest in the things that make me happy. Tearfulness – not sad-crying, but literally weeping all day, every day, at work, while running, upon waking, when going to sleep. I used to try and joke to my colleagues, 'I'm not really upset, this is just something my face is doing.' It was exasperating, but I couldn't stop it, or identify the cause.

The primary thing I look out for now is fatigue – a bone-deep exhaustion that no amount of sleep can lift. A few years ago, I was training for a 10k, relishing my fitness and stamina increasing run after run, when one day, my run through my local park felt different. It was a picture-perfect late autumn morning, like the world had made itself pretty just for me. I warmed up as usual, then fell into a steady trot. But somehow I didn't feel right. I wasn't sure how my legs worked, my arms seemed to be getting in my way, the path rose up too quickly and the balls of my feet jarred arrhythmically on the tarmac. Running felt like a language my body had never even heard of, let alone understood. I persevered, doggedly dragging one foot in front of the other, until I stopped. I should say: until my body made me stop. Every sinew and nerve in my throat, my shoulders, my forearms and my feet seized up, felt dark and heavy under my skin. My legs felt like lead. The best way I can describe it is that it was like instant flu. I collapsed on a bench for a while and sat in a daze, as the world continued to carry on with its day around me – prams were pushed, dogs were walked, babies were soothed. Then I crawled home and into bed and stayed there for three days. I told my boss I had the flu, but I didn't. There was no headache, fever, sore throat. Just insurmountable lethargy. I knew it was the onset of depression.

For those few days, I couldn't work. I hardly spoke to anyone.

I did nothing but eat, sleep and occasionally write down my thoughts. Self-care should be tangible, and when your brain stops working and nothing makes sense, what is tangible is profoundly comforting.

There are different levels of self-care you need to adopt at different times. Let's use a familiar analogy:

Adopt the traffic light system

GREEN
When everything seems hunky-dory, you still need to look after yourself to make sure things stay that way. Eat. Move. Sleep. Talk.

AMBER
When you're starting to feel noticeably stressed or unwell, do all of the above, and more. Stockpile good food in your home. Get admin jobs out of the way so you can focus on your needs. Be your own advocate. Ask for support where you can. Self-care can mean saying, 'This conversation/decision/ question is difficult for me at the moment. Can it wait until the end of the week?' It means setting boundaries and making space for yourself. Speak to your boss about managing your workload. If you have dependants, approach someone you trust and explain your situation. Gather your support network around you, even if it's very small. Just knowing people are there for you should you need to call on them will bring you peace of mind, and give you one less thing to worry about.

RED

All bets are off. Your first responsibility is to yourself, even if you have caring responsibilities – if you don't take care of yourself, there's a danger that you'll be less able to care for others. Seek medical advice. Call the Samaritans if you need to. Take some time off. Rally the troops – family, friends, loved ones. Eat. Communicate. Take your medication, if you have been prescribed it.

Plan your breakdown

A counsellor (not a shit one) once told me, 'If you feel as though you're about to have a panic attack – start planning it. Say you're on a busy train. Check how close you can get to the exit, so that you can disembark at the next stop. Plan how you'll ask that man to move his buggy so that you're closer to the exit. Consider where you'll put your coat if you need to lie down, where you'll put your bag. By accepting your anxiety rather than trying to suppress it, you'll find the feelings recede and you're less likely to have an attack.' By using this logic, you can minimise the impact of a potential breakdown by making space for your madness.

Make your environment as clean as you can. Empty the bins. Do the washing-up. Change your bedsheets and wash your favourite pyjamas. It sounds simple (maybe even condescending), but when you're ill, small stuff isn't small. When exhaustion kicks in, having the energy to do the most basic household tasks can feel impossible, and achieving something as simple as putting a load of laundry on can make a massive difference to the way you feel about yourself.

Write yourself a to-do list

When I was so ill I couldn't go to work, mine looked like this:

TO-DO LIST

* Get out of bed, shower, get dressed.
* Leave the flat for at least 30 mins a day.
* Cook dinner for my partner (I didn't care enough to cook for myself, but I'd cook for him). When I was single again I kept this habit going. Simple risottos, roast-in-a-bag chicken, pasta bakes. The writers Jack Monroe and Ruby Tandoh have some wonderful, easy, wholesome recipes for meals that cost very little to make and nourish your body and your heart.
* Order plenty of easy-prep, healthy-ish food to store, in case I'm not able to go to the shops.

NOT-TO-DO LIST:

* Go outside a two-mile radius of my home.
* Respond to emails if I didn't want to.
* Talk to anyone I didn't want to talk to.

Be kind to yourself. Your number one responsibility is to make yourself better. This can take time, and it's OK to opt out of the world to tend to your needs.

Build your support network

Talk to your friends and family about how you're feeling and let them help you – you'd do the same for them. If you have children or other dependants who rely on you, reach out to other parents, friends or neighbours. If they can't take time out from their own caring commitments to help you, look for help from a charity, a voluntary organisation or a professional carer. Remember the pre-flight safety demo you get on planes, when the flight attendant tells you to make sure you have sorted out your own life jacket and air supply before you help your child. It may feel wrong, but if you're not looking after yourself properly, you're not going to have the resources to care for others. Avoid carer burnout at all costs, as it will make navigating depression far more challenging.

Above all, ask for help

When I was ill, I was lucky enough to have a wonderful partner – he and my family were an amazing support network.

I turned to a number of experts, too: Samaritans, Mind and Rethink Mental Illness, to name a few. SANE's weekly texts (via Textcare) felt like a hand holding mine, and as the weeks went on they helped mark the passage of time – I was another week into my recovery, and further away from the truly awful first few days.

I think the most maddening thing – literally, the one thing that tips you from sanity to madness – is the cognitive dissonance, the disconnect between what you know as fact and what your mental illness is making you believe. You've got two or more trains of thought running in parallel with each other, contradicting each other, taking up the same amount of space in your brain. You may be able to see those negative thoughts for what they are – just thoughts – but you still have to experience them and feel them. And it's that presence – the constant, almost-physical weight of those spiralling thoughts that can stop me from sleeping. That's why I sometimes struggle to go out and reorder my medication and do the washing-up.

Luckily, in my case, I can always see the disparity between what I believe and what I know to be fact; I just can't turn off the bits that aren't fact. It seems to me that the bit of my brain that makes me creative and funny and smart and imaginative is the same bit that hurts me. And I haven't learned how to wrangle that yet.

I had my last panic attack about a year ago. I wrote:

> *My thoughts scurry like rats and there's no moderator, no impartial observer, no independent adjudicator, to go no of course your mam's not dead, of course your dad hasn't had a stroke, of course the job will be fine, and my brain won't shut up and fuck it's late. I'm a snake made mad by its own venom.*

I was pacing my bedroom, feeling the terror rising in my throat like a storm.

So I rang the number.

'Hello, Samaritans?' said a young-ish woman.

'Hello… I'm… having a… panic. Attack.'

'Oh, OK,' she said evenly. 'What normally helps with that?'

'Buh… brr… breathing.'

'OK. Why don't you try that now? Don't worry about talking. Just take your time.'

God, her voice was perfect. Smooth and steady, slightly concerned but not condescending, with all the right, predictable, sloping intonations: 'It's o-*kaaay*, take your *tiiime*, well *doooone*.'

I groped blindly for a towel, held it over my mouth, and scream-cried into it.

She told me her name was Hannah. This was probably a lie.

'It's o-*kaaay*, take your *tiiime*, well *doooone*. That's *gooood*.'

I came up for air, but kept the towel on hand to muffle my wailing. 'I feel like the worst person in the world but I know I'm not because I'm not a rapist or a murderer and I've never wilfully hurt anyone but I think I'm a horrible daughter and a burden to the people who love me…'

Out, out, out it rushed, all the bile in my head. No thought went unvoiced – money, relationships, my parents, my job, my friends, my body. How there was no milk in the fridge because I couldn't face the walk to the shops. How my eyes hurt because I hadn't reordered my contact lenses. On and on and on.

'And the thing is I can rationalise these thoughts and I can explain them away but they're still happening and I can articulate the difference between what I think and what I know but I can't switch those thoughts off I can't switch the feelings off and it still hurts it hurts *so much*.'

'OK.'

For about 40 minutes, I bawled until I was hoarse.

'Okaaaaay.'

'Thank you,' I hiccupped finally. 'I think I'm over the worst of it.'

'That's good. Well done. Is there anything else I can help you with?'

'No. Thank you, Hannah.'

'You're welcome. Call us back any time.'

I sat on my bed and texted my friend. *PA. Bad. 7/10. Called Samaritans. Over the worst.*

She replied in minutes. *Shit, mate. Have you slept? Is there food in?*

Slept OK. Extra-busy day today, so a bit anxious. Food in.

Excellent. Let me know how you feel in the morning. Love you. xx

I closed my eyes and took a few deep breaths. I felt a little light-headed, but the storm had passed. I got up, grabbed the soggy towel and headed for the shower.

Let someone else do one of your chores

If I really want to treat myself – I mean really push the boat out all the way – I don't go for a spa break or buy top-brand potions. To me, a service wash at a launderette is decadence bordering on the pornographic. It's expensive, but it's worth every penny to make your mouldy old gym kit, your heaps of bedding, your grotty damp towels, *someone else's problem.* You just hand it over and walk away, and you return a couple of days later to a pile of immaculately folded delights. You know how a sandwich tastes nicer when someone else has made it? Well, your clothes feel nicer when someone else has washed them. One fine day I might even upgrade to a collection service.

Write things down

I've said it before, but honestly, keeping track of your moods by writing them down is one of the cheapest and most effective things you can do for your mental health.

Here's another extract from one of my Depression Diaries:

Today was a nice day.
I washed all my clothes.

I tidied my room.

I ran.

I had my first shower in three days.

I drank lots of water, and took no sugar in my tea.

I drank a cup of green tea (FOUL).

I wrote a little.

I spent time on Instagram. I curled my hair.

I spoke to Ally and Mam and Dad.

I feel good. Now I'm going to mindfully brush my teeth and go to bed.

It's toe-curlingly dull, but that, to me, represents a corner being turned. Every single item on that list is an achievement, and one I was (and, fuck it, still am) proud of.

Now compare it to this extract from when I felt truly terrible:

I could sort out my tax.

I could arrange a cheaper phone contract.

I could apply for more jobs.

I could open the curtains.

I could wash and dress myself.

I could wash some clothes.

I could wash the dishes.

I could ring Mam and Dad.

I could go for a walk.

I could check out the gym timetable.

I could brush my teeth.

I could eat.

I could stay in bed (a very attractive option).

I could check my emails again just in case.

I could tidy up.
I could take some pictures.
I could write something.
But I don't want to do any of those things. I don't think I can.
So I think I'll just sit here.

When I feel really bad, I look at these lists. They're a reminder of how bad I have felt, and how far I've come.

Exercise

I know I keep banging on about it, and nobody ever *wants* to go running, but I find it works. For me, running is an act of self-love. I feel good after running, and not just because of the smugness – after years of pig-headed perseverance, the fabled endorphins have finally turned up, making my nerves crackle and my breath feel silky and cool in my lungs. It feels like power.

The art that saved my life

When your brain is made of despair, loneliness and fear, it's important to reacquaint it with joy, hope and human connection. That's what art is for. I was a huge bookworm as a kid and to this day, reading is one of my greatest pleasures. The cruellest thing about depression was that it robbed me of that ability. My concentration was in tatters. I was unable to access that pleasure and comfort when I needed it most.

So instead of reading prose, I started reading poetry and graphic novels. Work by Mariko Tamaki, Craig Thompson, Karrie Fransman, Dash Shaw, Neil Gaiman, Adrian Tomine,

Bryan and Mary Talbot; graphic reimaginings of classics, like the Sherlock Holmes graphic novel series by Ian Edginton and I N J Culbard, or the works of Alan Moore, Will Eisner and Art Spiegelman. I was already a fan, but when I was ill they became even more significant to me – looking at pictures interspersed with text was easier on my eye and brain, and the stories and illustrations nourished me like warm soup. I honestly credit the medium with my recovery, and these books continue to be an important part of my ongoing self-care practice.

Craig Thompson's illustrations are captivating at just the right frequency for my brain when it's depressed – they're intricate, but not hurt-your-eyes busy. His stories are heartfelt, but simple and linear. They soothed me.

Neil Gaiman's *Sandman* series, although at times too dark for my newly sensitive disposition, was great because I could finish a book in a day – which, when you're too depressed to shower or eat, feels like a significant, tangible achievement.

Find comfort where you can. Some people find it in baking. Others watch videos of corgis on YouTube. You don't have to understand what makes you feel good. You just have to allow yourself to enjoy things. One of the things that helped me more than I can fathom is a clip from the film *24 Hour Party People*, where a homeless man played by Christopher Eccleston recites from Boethius's *The Consolation of Philosophy*, which the ancient philosopher wrote in prison in AD524:

> *It's my belief that history is a wheel. 'Inconstancy is my very essence,' says the wheel. 'Rise up on my spokes if you like, but*

don't complain when you're cast back down into the depths.
Good times pass away, but then so do the bad. Mutability is
our tragedy, but it's also our hope. The worst of times, like the
best, are always passing away.'

'The worst of times, like the best, are always passing away.'
Isn't that something?

I love Rudyard Kipling's 'If—'. Always the same lines,
always the same videos and songs and poems. The repetition,
the sameness, made it easier for me to access the powerful
messages of resilience and hope that these artists have gifted
to us with their work.

Last year I took myself on a date for one. (I bloody LOVE
a date for one.) I went to the theatre to see *The Ferryman* by
Jez Butterworth. I'd booked the only ticket I could afford at
the time, a vertiginously remote nose-bleeder of a seat with a
severely restricted view. An almost entirely restricted view, in
fact. I asked the usher very nicely if I could upgrade, should
another seat at the theatre became available.

'It's sold out, so it's not likely, I'm afraid,' she said apologetically.

'Oh, I understand that,' I said, briefly wondering whether
I should flirt with her. I'm not very good at flirting – I'm
either far too subtle or far, FAR too not-subtle, so I went with
cheerful nonchalance. 'But I'm on my own, so if there was just
one spare seat anywhere at all with a better view, then I'd be
happy to take it.'

As we stood in the foyer with punters streaming around us
to their eye-poppingly expensive seats in the stalls, she assessed
me – a quick look up and down – before nodding approvingly.
'I can't promise anything, but I'll see what I can do.'

'Thank you so much.' I cracked a face-splitting smile at her and hoped for the best.

I crowbarred myself into my horrible seat and waited. Just as the lights dimmed, I felt a hand on my shoulder. It was her, the usher.

'There's standing room at the back of the stalls,' she said. 'It's a much better view, if you don't mind being on your feet.'

Joy swept through me. So I WAS good at flirting!

'Thank you so much,' I beamed again, as I grabbed my bag and raced downstairs to join the other dozen or so with standing tickets. I folded my coat over my arm and planted my feet just behind seats that cost ten times what I'd paid for mine. And I promise you, I had the best view in the house. The play, the writing, the *story*, was gorgeous. It curled up in my soul like a kitten and soothed me like nothing else had for a very long time. By the end of the first half, I was *drunk* on it.

I didn't move during the interval and shot evil eyes at anyone who came near me, stoutly standing my ground.

Just before the play started up again, I heard a crew member whispering to other people in the standing spaces. I fixed my eyes on the stage. If she was coming to claim the space that I had taken, I would NOT move. (Well, I would, obviously. I'm British. But I would give her *such* a filthy look when I did so. That'd teach her.)

Then she came to me.

'Are you on your own?' she whispered.

'Yes,' I answered warily.

'I'm the assistant director, and I have to leave now. So you can have my seat, OK?'

She pressed her ticket into my hand. I scanned it. Row H. Just eight rows from the stage.

'Oh my God,' I stammered, genuinely quite overcome.

I shook her hand (I can get weirdly formal when I'm emotional), she flashed a pretty smile before taking her leave, and I trotted over to claim my new seat.

I watched Paddy Considine in the lead role. He's one of the artists whose work helped me to get better. When I was very, very ill, I watched *Tyrannosaur*, the first film that he wrote and directed (a beautifully bleak film, but an unorthodox choice when you're severely depressed; you might as well include it in a triple bill, with *Requiem for a Dream* and *Schindler's List*). In the DVD extras, Paddy explained that, before writing the feature-length script, he'd written a four-minute film entitled *Dog Altogether*. I didn't think I could write a feature film, but at the time I thought I might be able to write a short one. I couldn't – turns out it's really, really hard – but it gave me something to focus on, and work towards, and wish for.

After the show, I popped into the pub opposite the theatre to have a quiet moment to myself before catching the Tube home. I'd just experienced something that was so earthy and rich and ALIVE, that made me pause and be thankful that I was better. I could see how far I'd come, and how much lighter and brighter my life was; more than I would have dared imagine back then. The chasm between how I had felt then and how I felt now was wide open before me, and it was all I could do not to fall on my fucking knees in gratitude that I'd made it out alive.

I can't credit Paddy Considine exclusively with my recovery.

Drugs have helped too. But art, and artists, have given me a reason to get better.

Does art alleviate my depression? Or is it a mere consolation?

I think both. There's no doubt that books like Marian Keyes's novel *Sushi for Beginners* have made me feel less alone. And I'm sure the cognitive exercise of reading, following a narrative and perceiving colours and shapes outside of the four walls of my flat, would scientifically benefit a broken brain. Isn't it marvellous that something so wonderful is actually good for you?

It's important to look at things that other humans have made. Other humans like you. Same brain, same elementary components, similar experiences. They make things that reflect those experiences and when it's done right, it feels like they've reached into your mind, pulled out a string of thoughts and are showing them to you – 'Look! That's you, that is!'

* * *

What art has helped you recover from an illness, a break-up or a bereavement?

Lara

Watching ballet. The immense beauty of it touches
and comforts me beyond almost anything else.

Amber

Dancing naked on stage at the Barbican in London in Nic
Green's *Trilogy* was pretty major! Completely changed my
relationship with my body.

Damian

That's an easy question, because I love them: the movie *I Kill Giants*, the graphic novel character Johnny Hiro and the *Beyond* anthology.

Amy

Good Morning, Midnight by Jean Rhys. Deeply sad but oddly comforting. I read it over and over.

Nicholas

Cricket is a comfort blanket for me

I read a lot of cricket books, huddled up on my bed reading about sporting feats and personalities from 100 years ago. Jack Hobbs, Sydney Barnes, Victor Trumper, Clem Hill, Ranji Hordern and Warwick Armstrong became my friends while I was far away from my real ones. I love cricket, there is something about the terminology and the way people write about it which is a comfort blanket for me. Some people dive into Philip K Dick or chocolate. I read about cricket, it feels like a secret language you need years of research to decipher. It also serves as a reminder than even niche figures can be remembered.

* * *

Self-harm

We all have a basic working knowledge of 'bad' coping mechanisms, whether it's drinking too much, taking recreational drugs or having sex with inappropriate partners. After a particularly grim episode, I made the decision to remove a lot of harmful coping mechanisms and to create healthy habits.

I would exercise.

I would eat well.

I stopped drinking.

I stopped working in a pub, to remove myself from bad influences.

And I stopped dating, vowing to stay single for a year.

I had come to realise that, for me, dating was another coping mechanism – a distraction – and I wanted to protect myself from the emotional upset of a short-lived relationship.

All these mechanisms do is help us avoid pain. And when we avoid pain, I believe that we avoid healing and recovery and growth.

So I know all about bad coping mechanisms. But what no one tells you – the crushing disappointment, the absolute shitter – is that there's no such thing as a perfect one.

Even after adopting healthy habits, all the anger, pain, grief, anxiety, sadness and exhaustion that I'd tried to avoid was still there waiting for me to process it, like a ton of backed-up jobs in a faulty printer. Now they were coming to the surface, like farts in a swamp.

I couldn't reason with them.

When you have depression, you're aware of it all the time.

You get into bed with it and fall asleep with it heavy on your chest.

It's there every weekend when you call your parents.

It's there when you ask your sister what to get your niece for her birthday.

It's there when your boss praises your work.

It's there when you style your hair and do your make-up.

It's there at dinner with friends.

It's there when you go on a date.

So, when there's an opportunity for distraction, a little bit of oblivion, a drink or a cigarette or a meandering text exchange, is it any wonder you cling to these opportunities to escape your own horrible thoughts like a life jacket?

Another lie you tell yourself: you will convert your pain into something useful, maybe even beautiful.

Nope.

While you can channel your suffering, you can't remove it. It's not something you can draw out of yourself until it's all gone forever, like a tapeworm. You can talk about having a toothache, but it doesn't cure the toothache. Talking about mental and emotional pain is useful, and it relieves the burden of shame. But you can't out-think your own feelings. They don't dissolve when you finally understand them. You don't stop feeling them just because you can rationalise them. That's why I've only ever been disappointed by those meditation apps. I used them thinking they'd help me opt out of my pain for ten minutes. But they don't. Of course they don't. I know that the purpose of meditation is to learn to live with and observe my feelings more objectively, and I'd like to learn how to do that. But first I have to not want to obliterate them.

Why I don't like meditation

I'm going to tell you about a very strange thing that happened the only time that I actually meditated properly. And of all the weird and intimate and deeply embarrassing events in my life so far, this is the one I'm most reluctant to share. Because this is one of the few one-off events that have happened in my mind that I'm actually, genuinely afraid of.

As anyone who's ever talked openly about their mental health will tell you, this is the question they're asked most often:

'Have you tried meditation?'

I *had* tried meditation, but I just couldn't do it, I thought, in the same way that some people can't roll their tongue, or aren't double-jointed. My brain just won't *bend* that way.

And to prove it, I signed myself up for a two-day meditation workshop, on the recommendation of someone I was working in a pub with at the time.

The workshop took place over a weekend in the assembly room of a primary school just around the corner from where I live. The leader – a very kind man in his 40s – was perched at a table, happily chatting away to a couple of people he seemed to know. He gave me a smile and a nod, which I returned while trying not to audibly gag when I saw what was on the table in front of him: a singing bowl. And *crystals* – loads of them, in different colours and shapes that I was certain had *meanings* and *properties* I'd be lectured about. I eyed the fire exit longingly, but before I could scuttle away, the nice man introduced himself, told me I was very welcome, and that he hoped I'd have a lovely weekend. The *bastard*.

Fine, I thought grimly. *But if anyone mentions chakras, I'm off.*

The first thing we did was an exercise where we had to get into pairs and maintain eye contact in silence for seven minutes. *Seven. Minutes.* I was matched with, objectively, the most handsome boy there, which made me deeply uncomfortable. How was I supposed to connect my flawed emotional mechanics with a boy I'd be too scared to talk to in a pub? But I did it. Seven minutes of eye contact, in total silence. When it was over, we were invited to discuss our experience with our partner. I was feeling pretty chuffed with myself. First exercise: nailed. Turned out I was BRILLIANT at being a hippy. Maybe I *DID* have chakras. 'Err, thank you,' I stammered. 'I've never done anything like that before. I felt you were quite committed and non-judgemental, although I was quite uncomfortable at first.'

He nodded. God, he seemed so *wise*, like a sexy but spiritual lumberjack. Had I finally found the spot where all the wise, emotionally together people hung out? Was I one of them now?

Just as I was contemplating getting a singing bowl of my own, he spoke. 'I felt nothing. I've done this plenty of times, and I wasn't uncomfortable. I mean…' he gestured impatiently at my face, '…they're just eyes. It didn't really bring anything up for me. It was like looking into a black void.'

Ah. Not a shaman, more of a shithead.

Silent meditation is dangerous. You can project all kinds of wonderful qualities on to people before they open their mouths.

He left shortly after that.

The next exercise was to 'connect with your inner critic' by making a list of our flaws. This would be easy! I enthusiastically started making my list – undisciplined, childish, self-absorbed, defensive, crap with money, work-shy, blah blah blah. I felt quite smug, my long-dormant proclivity for being a teacher's pet coming to the surface. I was going to be the BEST at hating myself. I was in my element.

To my horror, we were then directed to get into groups

(urgh) and actually *read out loud* our litany of flaws. And then again, this time in the style of a film noir femme fatale. Then in the style of Veruca Salt from *Charlie and the Chocolate Factory*. Then a porn star. Then a high court judge. Over and over again, in fact, until the whole group dissolved into fits of giggles and those words – those spiteful, poisonous barbs we'd been torturing ourselves with – lost all power to hurt us. The most shameful, frightening ideas my brain could produce were now themselves the subject of mirth, as I snorted and yelped my way through the list with tears of laughter streaming down my cheeks.

Next, we were asked to share our most shameful memory.

Oooh. This one hurt. And it still hurts.

It happened when I was working in Edinburgh. I was gluing reviews to posters in torrential rain. Edinburgh is one of my favourite places in the world, but it's a city that could have been built by Escher. Everything is cobbled, every direction is uphill, and it's always, always raining. I saw a wheelchair user nearby who appeared to need some help to navigate the uneven path and get to a venue, but I had to glue reviews to posters. So that's what I kept doing, instead of offering to help him. In the end, he asked a passer-by. And I was so disgusted with myself that I snuck into the backstage area of one of the theatres and sobbed my heart out.

I was so desperate to be good at my job that I'd acted against what I knew to be the right thing to do. What I'd been brought up to do. I imagined my parents and my sisters – an ambulance technician, a carer for the elderly and two SEN teachers – being appalled and ashamed of me. Even now, the memory of my selfishness makes me itch with shame.

I shared this with the group, and there was no judgement. That was nice. I didn't feel any better, but it did make me realise that carrying shame isn't always useful. I walked home that night feeling good, and settled. I slept restfully, and awoke refreshed and ready for the next session the following day.

Which is where it gets... weird.

Here's the exercise. You close your eyes, and imagine yourself sitting in a chair next to a bookshelf. In your mind, you take down a book, write your name in it, and place it back on the shelf. You take down a second book, and write everything you've ever said and done, every life experience, and place it back on the shelf. In the third book, you write everything you've ever thought and felt, and place it back on the shelf. Finally, you take a fourth book, write everything you've ever learned, and place it back on the shelf. Now, in theory, you are to examine what's left. After you've removed everything you've ever said and done, everything you've ever thought and felt, everything you've ever learned, and all the arbitrary stuff about you – your name, your nationality, the number of years you've been alive – what's left?

Having stripped away every conscious experience of my life, I could see what else I *was* made of.

What was left was a ball of white light. It was... apparently *there*, in front of me. True, it was in my mind's eye, but it was still... there, shockingly real and present and palpable. My eyes still closed, I shifted in my chair to face it, and in doing so I saw more and more balls of white light, one in front of each person in the room and beyond, in Bristol, in the South

West, in the UK, in the world. And these balls of white light were connected, and they were all the same. And I was overwhelmed by a sense of empathy, but more than empathy. Empathy *squared*. I'm not *like* them, I *am* them, and they are me, and we are all this ball of white light. And then I realised that I was outside of my own body. I was actually inside the white light. The word BENEVOLENCE resounded in my head, behind my eyes. I felt happy, *overwhelmed* with happiness. I placed my hand over my heart and sat still for a very long time.

When my awareness came back, and I opened my eyes, I was exhausted, I felt like I'd occupied a psychic space that I'd never occupied before, like I'd opened a door in my brain and found a new room that had always been there. And I wasn't sure that I was better off knowing about it. It felt like some sketchy hippy shit that scared the hell out of me. I don't know how the crystals were involved, but they definitely were somehow, the shady little pricks. And I don't want it to happen again.

And that's why I don't meditate.

* * *

Self-care is hard. How do other people do it? I asked them: what does self-care look like to you?

Catie
I used my photographs to reach out to people

After losing both parents within six months of one another, my mental health spiralled, but I ignored it.

I locked up all that sadness and anger deep inside and pretended it didn't exist. I refused to talk about what had happened, believing that's what it meant to be strong. It wasn't until I started a university project almost ten years later that I realised just how bad my mental health was. I would sleep in late, ignore daily life, struggle with emotions, tell people I had other plans so I didn't have to go out and face them, and my self-worth and confidence were at an all-time low. I hated myself. I was lost and feeling hopeless.

A lecturer of mine had used photography as a kind of therapy, which opened a completely new door to me. I could use this, I could attempt to heal.

I used my photographs to reach out to people, to speak through imagery about my losses in an attempt to help others, but also as catharsis.

That decision completely changed my approach to mental health, as it was no longer taboo to speak about the dark things in my mind, they were no longer something to be ashamed of. The fact that my parents had passed away was now not something people could pity me for, but something they could relate to. I'm not saying that I'm 100 per cent cured, I never will be, but I can manage. There will always be dark days where I miss them so much my heart aches. On these days, I look at photographs of them and remember that they taught me to live my life, they raised me wonderfully, I had an amazing childhood filled with so much love and laughter. The people around me have given me strength to carry on. They are the pillars of my being, without whom I would not be here today.

Julia
*You have to take time for yourself, even if it's
15 minutes a day*

As a parent, it's important to ask for help, reframe the guilt and shame and remember that if you're not OK, your kids aren't OK. You have to plan to take time for yourself, even if it's 15 minutes a day at first, and devote every one of those minutes only to yourself. The more you make yourself a priority, the easier it will become!

Sally Marie
I listen to audiobooks during chores

I've got a 12-year-old autistic son who is at home 24/7 (home tutored, as he can't cope with school) and a four-year-old who has just started school. I try and fit in little things that make me happy during the day. Today I treated myself to my favourite bagel on the way home from the school run – it gave me something to look forward to when I was sobbing over the dishwasher. When I'm down I'll leave a chore (usually washing up!) for later and watch one of my comfort TV shows, like *Parks and Recreation* or *Pride and Prejudice* for an hour. I also listen to audiobooks during chores – it stops my rampant self-loathing and anxiety from crowding my brain during otherwise mindless tasks.

Anonymous
My therapy is his future

I've struggled with depression my whole life. I'm now 50 and have one child who is almost 16. The day he was born, my whole world changed. My therapy is his future. I want to see him grow into a fine young man. I still get blue now and then, but I pray for strength. Thank goodness for my supportive husband, too – I would be lost without him.

Gregg

If you're anxious about making a decision, eat a snack first

Part of knowing who you are and becoming the best person you can be is to take ownership of yourself, and that includes the good and the bad things. And the more you have mastery over your own emotions, the more you feel in control of your own life and what's going on. Part of anxiety and depression is feeling hopeless; things are happening *to* you, and you're just reacting. So the more you build yourself up and respect the person you are, the easier self-care gets. You've got to look at yourself as a person you like and a person you want to help. So treat yourself like you would someone you love and want to look after. The more you do it, the more positive outcomes happen.

Be aware of your mood in a situation, and start from as calm a place as possible before you make a decision. Just stop, take a few breaths in and out, and then decide. This is a really small and simple thing, but if you're anxious about it, eat a snack first. It can really help.

I meditate. Five to ten minutes every morning, just to start the day with a calm brain. I'm making an effort to have less screen time, so I try not to watch stuff before bed.

Exercise helps, because physical tension affects your allostatic load (the wear and tear on your physical body that affects your stress hormones). It's a catch-22, so you have to calm your body and your mind down at the same time. I hate running, but I do it. Your frame of mind definitely has an effect on your physical body, like a feedback loop.

Sol

When I'm high, I make my plans for when I'm low

I get lows and highs. When I'm high, I make my plans for when I'm low, to pick myself up. I see friends. I design menus. I make plans for my own company. And I take one weekend a month to go away with my husband and my younger son. We pack up a van, go by the sea, go fishing. In the middle of my own depression, I can see I don't want to be depressed. Yes, I can't stop crying. But at the same time, I know I don't want to be like that forever. So, when I'm high, I start planning and looking for the next thing that'll make me better. Your family is counting on you, so be there for them.

I suppose after 25 years of ups and downs, I have to trust myself. Beautiful people have helped me on the way. In the middle of all the crying and the smiles, they're still there.

9

My Shit Home

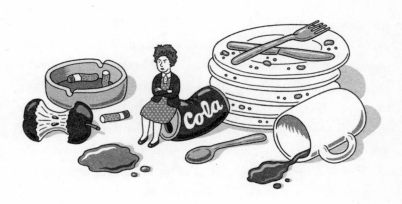

I HAVE MOVED HOUSE 14 TIMES IN 12 YEARS.
I was desperate to leave home the minute I turned 18. I have a wonderful family, but I had no friends and no job prospects. In my home town, there was a pyjama factory, a chocolate factory that I worked in for two summers as a student, and a bakery. None of them were hiring.

My parents knew I was dying to move away, so they helped me. I couldn't have done it without them. My first home from home was a tiny little flat in an armpit of a village with a train station, between Wrexham and Chester.

Since then I've lived in house-shares, dorms, spare rooms and on sofas. Twice I've lived through a strange, limbo-ish 'you-can-crash-at-mine-for-a-bit' situation with boyfriends.

According to UK property website Zoopla, the average person in the UK moves eight times in their life. But with many millennials graduating during or just after the 2008 crash, then having to move to find work, many have had a similar experience to me. Today only one in five of my generation has the means to put down roots by buying their own home. What's that doing to our well-being?

Recently the mental health charity Mind launched a major housing campaign, with figures showing that nearly 79 per cent of people with mental health problems say a housing situation has either caused that problem or made it worse.

'Housing and mental health are often linked,' says Paul Spencer, a policy manager at Mind. 'The lack of security in rented accommodation can be damaging for mental health, and involuntary home moves can have a particularly severe effect... It may also mean you have to move away from mental health services or other services in your community that were supporting you.'

It's not just the financial aspect of where you live that can affect your mental health and sense of well-being. Home isn't just four walls and a roof. It's a sanctuary. It's somewhere you can retreat to and feel safe in. And when that doesn't feel secure or, worse, when it's suddenly taken away, nothing feels right.

The party house

I once lived in the classic party house where everyone ended up after a night out. My room was on the ground floor, next to the living room, where the unemployed stoner would play Seasick Steve on a loop all night, and underneath the Spanish DJ whose mates would pile in gurning at 5am and blast Hot Chip while singing along: 'DOBER AN DOBER AN DOBER AN DOBER AN DOBERRRRRR.' Every night was an aural spit-roast.

The headquarters-of-a-cult house

When I first landed in London, I lived in a gorgeous, huge Victorian house. I could see the O2 from my room, which *thrilled* me. I was living with three other girls, but we rarely exchanged a word. It was as though I'd accidentally moved into a convent where everyone had taken a vow of silence. People left passive-aggressive notes if there were crumbs on the kitchen table. Even though there was a spacious kitchen – massive by London standards – each of them kept their own pots and pans in their room. At mealtimes they'd bring them out, cook with headphones in without talking to each other, wash up, then *take everything back to their rooms*. At first it was a minor quirk that I could put up with for an affordable room. After a few months, it was unbearable.

There was (of course) a rota for cleaning and buying toilet paper. I once missed my turn for buying toilet paper because I was on tour for three weeks. When I returned, I was confronted in the kitchen by one of the women.

'You miss your turn to buy toilet paper,' she rasped.

'Yes,' I said nicely. 'I wasn't here.'

'We are without toilet paper for three weeks.'

Christ alive.

'What have you done before when this has happened?'

'It never happens before,' she announced.

'How… how long have you lived here together?'

'Me, seven years. The others, five.'

This chilled me. The house was quiet and cheap, and I had a huge room in a fantastic location, but I only lasted six months. It was as creepy as it was desperately sad that three people would willingly isolate themselves from those they shared a home with.

The house that ended a friendship

I moved in with a friend who I loved dearly, but I soon saw a side of him that I'd never seen before. His ego was astounding. He bragged about how much money he had (when we all knew he was borrowing from another housemate to make rent). He stockpiled dirty dishes in his room. To my surprise and disappointment, he was also disgustingly misogynistic. How had I not seen that before? Thankfully, the other housemate stopped bankrolling him and he had to move back in with his mum.

The house that went off

I lived in a place with such profound damp that when I went to grab a pair of shoes from my wardrobe, I discovered they'd disintegrated with mould.

The house that got awkward

I lived with a couple. A few weeks in, I found the man's profile on a dating site, marked ACTIVE. I never told her and I didn't confront him. I'm not sure whether I regret that or not.

The arthaus

This was a spectacularly beautiful artist's house, all Farrow & Ball paint and colour-coded crockery and exquisite ceramics. My live-in landlady had spent so much money making her home painfully beautiful that she now had to share it with lodgers to cover her mortgage, something she clearly resented. I was warned not to put anything too hot on the ruinously expensive worktops. She would take my washing down when it was still damp because it 'took up too much room' in the kitchen. The empty bottle of booze and baggies of class A drugs that she left lying around were apparently fine, though. Much more aesthetic than soggy pyjamas.

The house that was home

Once upon a time I lived with a boy in a flat that we filled with love and laughter, until the day came when I cried in the stairwell and left forever.

A few weeks later I received my decree absolute. We hadn't been married so this was the millennials' version, an email confirming that the deposit I'd paid on the flat I'd once shared with my ex-partner in my longest relationship so far had finally been refunded.

A lot had happened between the end of that relationship and receiving the email. Life had gone on. As Boethius reminded us, 'Good times pass away, but then so do the bad.' But this notification, this cold scrap of legal data, served as a reminder that something fundamental had shifted. I'd changed something. Failed at something. Lost something I'd never have again.

* * *

After I moved out, I spent three weeks on friends' sofas before finding a tiny box-room five minutes away from what had been my (our) lovely little flat. There was so much guilt, so much doubt, so much anger and self-loathing. There was some little relief, too, streaking through the tumult like angel rays. But aside from the grief – the terrible, corrosive grief that contaminated every aspect of every day and left me reeling (ever stuck your head in a fridge to hide a fresh batch of tears from your colleagues? I have), there was a nauseating amount of financial admin and paperwork involved. Separating our belongings, working out how to get to work from my mate's place on the night bus, changing my address on bills and statements (this particularly tedious bit of ball-achery took me six months to complete).

There was a hefty price to pay, too – removal vans to hire, greater commuting costs, a deposit and a month's rent in advance on my new place as well as a month's final rent on my former home. It was dizzying and frightening and now I know why people stay in unhappy relationships and marriages. Especially parents – I can't imagine doing all that while caring for a small, scared child – I myself felt like a small, scared child. I called my mam and dad constantly, unable to make the smallest decision without consulting them. I was fortunate enough to have their infinite patience and love.

The flat deposit was the final thread connecting me to my ex – the refund signified that he had finally moved out of what had once been our home.

When the relationship ended, my anxiety flared up like psoriasis but I had no outlet. I couldn't ask him if he was all right because I knew that he wasn't. I knew that I was the reason he wasn't all right, and I felt sick with guilt because I still loved him. I'd broken his heart but I still loved him so much. My friends and family carried me through those frightful few weeks. They spoke soothing words and rubbed my back when I had panic attacks in the pub. They didn't flinch when I snotted and slobbered all over them like a rabid mastiff. They protected me when I was hurt, and they prevented me from hurting myself. Their love saved me. There have been a few times in my life when my self-esteem has shrivelled completely, and the one thing that has helped pull me through is a good look at the people who love me. I might not like myself sometimes, but *they* like me. I trust their opinion more than I trust my own, therefore I can't be all that bad. See? Even a depressed person can follow that logic.

I was very sad when my relationship ended, even grief-stricken, but I wasn't depressed. I didn't feel debilitated by the sadness – in fact, it was imbued with relief that it was over, that we were both free to pursue what we really wanted from life. It seemed that this relationship had reached a point where I had to choose between my partner or myself. And I chose myself.

It took a long time to acclimatise to my single status. My husband (we were never married, but I always called him that, even at the very beginning) had been my compass. Now I was adrift and I couldn't tell dry land from stormy sea. I even started smoking again. Our relationship, my life's anchor, had been re-examined and reclassified, and there's so much more to that than no longer sharing a roof. It's a rending of the soul. It hurts. I was so lonely. I was so lost, and I had lost so much. But it was still time to leave.

For a long time, every time I had to catch a train, I had to walk past our old home. His car wasn't parked outside anymore, and there were new curtains and shiny new furniture in the back room (of course I still looked, every time). I still had a sense of this place representing a line between my new life and one where we were still together, between the present and the past. But then I'd catch my train in my new present. In my new place. In my new world.

* * *

Where we live has a fundamental influence on our sense of well-being, but finding a secure home to make your own can be far harder if you are struggling with depression. How does where you live affect your mental health?

Nicholas
I registered as homeless

During a particularly bad time I was unable to fully relax or feel safe for a year. First, I moved into a flat, owned by a man who neglected to mention that he would enjoy coming into my room when I was asleep, espousing extreme political views and occasionally becoming physically and verbally aggressive. I did not have the money to find another place: so when he broke the locks and forced his way into the flat and threatened me, I called the police. They informed me (when they arrived three days later) that since it was his flat and he was not a registered landlord and the flat wasn't HMOed, he could legally come in whenever he liked. So I registered as homeless and I was moved into a converted old people's home in Easterhouse in Glasgow. I was there for four months. I am not sure if I felt nuts because of the situation or because of my predisposition to depression and anxiety, but it wasn't a fun time.

Shona
I moved 300 miles from home to be with someone I loved

I didn't realise the impact it would have on my mental health. I felt totally isolated without my friends and family and ended up back on the medication I'd come off.

How to be alone but not lonely

When I was in my last miserable house-share, I knew it had to be my last. I had to find somewhere where I could live alone. I imagined a tiny studio with lots of light, a desk where I could write. Room for my books. I longed for it. I dreamed about it. And, miraculously, I found it. My kitchen has an oven, a fridge (no freezer) and two cupboards, but I can cook elaborate meals for myself with a glass of something delicious and feel like the person I was always meant to be. You can't commandeer the kitchen for four hours in a house-share. Not everyone wants to listen to a grimly graphic true-crime podcast while they're whipping up a snack (weirdos). I occasionally worry about my neighbours' children overhearing a particularly grisly episode of *My Favourite Murder* (but not enough to turn it down). And while I don't think I'm in my forever home, if I stay where I am for more than a year, it'll be a welcome change.

However, when you live alone, and everyone you know is busy with kids/work/Netflix, sometimes you have to force yourself to socialise to stop going full *Cast Away*. And that means stepping out on your own on a date for one, a solo mission, like a spy or a grizzled old detective or Amélie, from the film by Jean-Pierre Jeunet, before that horrible old man puts a massive, unsolicited downer on her fabulous single life.

You have to find the right venue – a cosy cafe in an art gallery, a cocktail place where no one knows you and you can stand at the bar and try on a new identity. A nice pub will do. I used to live near a Wetherspoon's that was so vast and labyrinthine I could always find a teeny little corner table and hide with a book and a very reasonably priced G&T. Little local indie pubs where the staff are friendly enough for a natter if that's what you fancy, but polite enough to leave you in peace if you don't, are cool, too.

At Meetup.com you can set up a group for your activity and invite others to join, whether it's mass dog walks, trips to the theatre or spoken word nights. I've set myself a goal to do more fun stuff with more new people. Trampoline dodgeball? Sure! Axe-throwing? Why not? Bouldering? No, that looks hard. A group for people who think men who describe themselves as 'cheeky chappies' on their dating profiles belong on a register? Sign. Me. Up.

Where do you meet new people when you have a mental health problem?

One option is a mental health support group. Also known as group therapy, or peer-to-peer counselling.

When I was ill, all those years ago, I couldn't stand the thought of being part of a group of depressed strangers talking about how depressed they were. I didn't think I could bear the weight of anyone else's pain, and I felt too fragile to express mine so publicly.

But I'd moved cities since then, and the landscape of my life had shifted so dramatically it was almost unrecognisable. I was well, and I wanted to stay well, and finding out how other people got and stayed well made sense. I rolled the idea around in my mind like a boiled sweet. And one Tuesday in October, just after the clocks changed, I turned up in a draughty church rectory for my very first mental health support group meeting.

It was half-full when I arrived (which meant there were around five people present. It was a very snug rectory). I walked in from the cold to see a smiling woman chatting to another and making a coffee, while two cyclists good-naturedly negotiated space for their bikes.

I'd felt fine about going alone (after texting my friends for moral support). It felt like a little adventure, a new experience. Who would I meet? Anyone I knew? Would there be BOYS? (Although surely it would be a catastrophically awful idea to get romantically involved with someone I met at a mental health support group. Wouldn't it? Probably. Yes, definitely, I almost certainly won't do that then. Most likely.) What I hadn't considered was how walking through that door would make me feel about myself. I felt terribly vulnerable, and awfully, awfully alone. I loitered by the door, tears pricking my eyes, when I caught the eye of the smiling woman who was making coffee – the group leader.

'Shall we pop next door?' she said diplomatically, and ushered me into the next room.

'I was a mess at my first session,' she continued sympathetically, as I sniffed and tried to get my bottom lip under control. 'I didn't share anything with the group for weeks. It's OK. There's no pressure. And everyone here knows exactly how you're feeling.'

I felt very… *young*, all of a sudden. Childlike and desperate for comfort, for a grown-up to tell me everything was going to be all right.

I thanked her, and we headed back into the main room, and the session began. I sat on an empty sofa and prayed that no one would sit next to me. I had wanted a chair, my own demarcated space, but they were all snapped up. I kept my eyes on the floor.

I didn't want to risk eye contact. A kind smile would almost certainly set me off again.

The seat next to me was taken, extra chairs were unstacked, sofas rearranged ('Mind the bikes!'). The gender split was pretty even, and there was a wide age range, from students to retirees.

It was freezing cold, and I wished I'd made myself a hot drink while I'd had the chance.

At the beginning, the two facilitators read out the group rules.

No interrupting.

No offering advice unless asked.

No personal information about anyone not present.

No brand names for any medication.

Fake names were acceptable, as long as this was the same one used at every session you attended.

No biting (not really).

In the end, I didn't share anything. I didn't know what to say. And of course I'm not going to share anyone else's stories here.

But I realised that I had been wrong. Going to a mental health support group meeting wasn't depressing, even though some deeply upsetting thoughts and experiences were shared.

It was uplifting to hear people – ordinary people – speak candidly about their mental health in their own words. To hear them claim it, *own* it, say *my* bipolar, *my* addiction, *my* PTSD.

The only time I spoke was to join the group in saying, 'Thank you for sharing' when each person stopped speaking. It's such a cliché that we've all said it, ironically, like when someone tells us they're going for a wee. But that night I meant it from the bottom of my heart.

'Thank you for sharing.'

'Thank you for sharing.'

'Thank you for sharing.'

'Thank you for sharing.'

At the end of the session, attendants could set a goal if they chose to. Mine was to go back the following week. I didn't; life got in the way. But that's OK. And at some point I'll be ready to hear a roomful of people thank *me* for sharing.

A short nice thing that happened to me

I was moving out of the home where I had lived with my ex. I was alone, sitting among half-packed boxes. And I could feel my mental state slipping, hear the damning chorus gearing up between my ears. So I did what I always do. I phoned a friend – the mad boy I used to go out with.

'OK, Michelle,' he said. 'What are the voices saying?'

'That I've done this to myself. That I was born with something missing, I'll never be happy.'

I curled up on the floor and cried (it wasn't just for dramatic effect, the furniture was gone). And he listened and soothed and reassured me.

'We're all just toothless prospectors panning for happiness,' he announced. 'So shit on the voices, Michelle. You're great. And I love you.'

No one can cure your depression. But having one kind person who loves you tell it to fuck off can help a lot.

My Brilliant Shit Brain

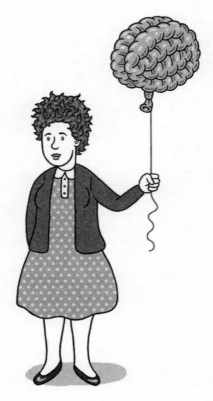

HAPPINESS AND SELF-ESTEEM CO-EXIST LIKE TWO gorgeous, romping Siberian huskies. One can't exist without the other – you must nurture both. Without enough self-esteem, we won't seek out happiness (because we feel we don't deserve it). If we're not happy, it may be because we don't value ourselves enough to begin to change our circumstances and pursue joy.

We only get one life; it's a sin to squander it on fear, bitterness and joylessness. The world has so many beautiful, smart, enriching things to fill your head and your heart: books, art, films, dancing, cooking, hiking, competitive spear fishing... Try *everything*. Start a band. Take photographs. Write a blog. Find out what you like and keep doing it, even if it's only for a couple of hours each week. Tend to your soul's needs, and the holistic benefits will filter through every aspect of your life, like sunbeams.

Low self-esteem can lead to us making harmful decisions in our career, in our friendships and in our romantic relationships. It is one of your duties in this life to make your own happiness, self-esteem and satisfaction a priority.

When I was very young, before I knew how big the world was and how many ways there were to be engaged, interested and fulfilled by it, I viewed my life as a barren landscape with a few flourishes of colour dotted along a distant horizon. I wanted to bypass the dull desert – literally to skip years of school and young adulthood – and get to the colourful, vibrant, exciting bit where *stuff* happened. I wanted to opt out of what I saw then as the monotonous, unfulfilling period of my life, and fast-forward. I realise now that that is a deeply depressive thought, but at the time I didn't see myself as being depressed. Sure, I was bored, isolated, unfulfilled and disempowered, but I assumed everyone else was, too. I didn't realise at the time how vitally important it is to be able to make your own fun, whatever your circumstances. And today, I know how to make my own fun, even in the desert. As much as my brain can be an asshole, it can also be a pretty cool place to live.

What are the best things about being batshit?

1. My mind is a fortress

    That's an exaggeration, but I'm a hell of a lot calmer, and very few things scare me since I've recovered from a mental illness. Public speaking? Bring it on. Tough deadline? Too easy. Getting dumped? Pah. It's like I've had my software upgraded after a malware attack, and now I've got a shitload of cool new features, like improved resilience and a robust sense of self.

2. My relationships are stronger

    Having depression has given me a much deeper appreciation for my family and friends. Now I'm better at tending to those relationships, and (hopefully) letting my loved ones know how much I appreciate them.

3. I'm more empathetic and compassionate than I used to be

    Having a crappy mental health day? I got you, dude. Want to chat antidepressants? Pull up a pew and let's get into it.

4. Recovering from my depression has proven to me that I am bigger than my depression

I used to believe the awful trope that you had to be miserable to make good art, but having depression has never made me creative. Depression just makes me depressed. Working hard at being creative makes me creative (most of the time). And when you conjure something into existence that wasn't there before using only your bare brain and hands and heart, it makes you feel a tiny bit invincible, and reminds you that you are more than your mental illness.

5. Problem-solving is my jam

I once met a man with a very severe stammer. One of the ways he managed his condition was by developing an extraordinarily broad vocabulary, so that he could avoid using his trigger words and sounds by using a synonym or changing the sentence structure. As a result, his speech patterns were nothing short of enthralling (he also had a soft Scottish accent, and was the most devastatingly well-dressed man I've ever met).

The point is that the method he used to master his stammer helped shape the person he became, and arguably was one of his biggest strengths.

I'm hoping that the steps I've taken to master and make friends with my depression make me a more interesting human, who's better equipped to deal with the curveballs that life will continue to throw at me.

6. I have never lost a phone, purse, bag or set of keys

Anxiety gets me to compulsively check my belongings every four minutes or so.

7. I'm fairly bomb-proof

    There is nothing anyone can say to me that I haven't already thought about myself, and either proven wrong, or forgiven myself for. Me and myself are pretty tight these days.

8. I know my limits

    Self-knowledge is a gift. I know my warning signs. I'm mindful of the tone I use when I'm talking to myself because I'm aware that I'm bad at self-compassion. If I know I have a busy period coming up at work, I'll take extra care to eat well, move more, schedule some quiet time and listen to my body and my mind.

Here's what others had to say in praise of being potty:

Lauren

I absolutely treasure the empathy I have as a result of struggling

I've been aware of my mind being... atypical most of my life. I've felt the challenges of mental illness keenly. I battle with taking my medications, because I genuinely love my brain.

I love the way I ponder issues because of my racing thoughts. I love my creativity. I am an artist and a musician, both mostly as hobbies. But most of all, I absolutely treasure the empathy I have as a result of struggling as I have. I think I value other people and appreciate them so hard, because I get it.

Harald
I can 'read' others more easily

I accept a kind of hypersensitivity within myself, which gives me the ability to 'read' others more easily, and the chance to show my unprotected soul to others. I am proud that I am who I am.

Nicholas
My self-destructive tendencies have led me on some weird adventures

It can be genuinely be fun not being able to trust your own mind or decisions (I'm referring to the times when my mental illness isn't debilitating and a fucking nightmare). My self-destructive tendencies have led me on some weird adventures.

Kerstin
We who suffer from a mental illness are just more sensitive and receptive to what is going on in our environment

I see my mental illness as a gift now. Sure, it's a gift that I wouldn't wish on anybody. But I know I am strong, and I have to be. My mission is to enjoy life just for the sake of it. I find peace in little things, mostly nature. I know that I need more me-time than most people. But I feel that life is just great, and that we who suffer from a mental illness are just more sensitive and receptive to what is going on in our environment. We can turn it into something good!

Gregg

*Not quite being connected to the world gives me angles that
other people don't have*

Having a weird brain makes me do weird stuff and have
niche interests. I like patterns and analysing things. I have a
different way of looking at the world. I get spaced out, I go off
on tangents. I've been doing political analysis. So I think not
being quite connected to the world gives me angles that other
people don't have.

The big, sexy ending

It's been six years since I went mad. I've been on medication
for four. And while (touch wood) my mental health is pretty
robust these days, there's a part of me, sure as a shadow, that
will always live in terror of losing my mind again. So if you're
feeling fragile, here's my advice from the other side of the
psychic shitshow:

* When you're in pain, allow yourself 15 minutes to
  do nothing. Go to bed if you can. Alternatively, put
  on some do-not-disturb headphones and find a quiet
  corner to take some deep breaths in.
* There is no reinventing the wheel when it comes to
  despair. I wish I'd known how wrong I was when
  I took my 15-year-old self to the doctor because I
  thought no one else felt the way I did. Just as there are
  12 musical notes and only seven stories in the world,
  there are a finite number of traumas that the human

psyche can experience. And each one – no matter how profound, debilitating or painful – has been met and overcome by another human just like you. It's true that there have been people who've felt unable to bear the burden that you're living with. But there are also others who have endured what may seem to be unendurable, and have survived what appears now to be insurmountable.

So please. All you need to do is to hold on, even when it hurts. Even when you're tired. Even when you're poor. Even when you're convinced that the people who love you would be better off if you let go.

Please hold on.

Please stay with us.

We need you.

Glossary

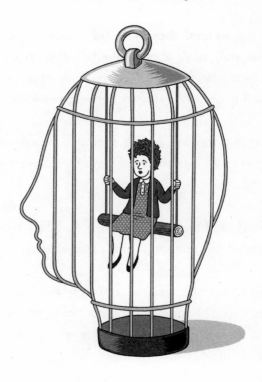

Antidepressants are thought to work by increasing the levels of chemicals in the brain called neurotransmitters. SSRIs (selective serotonin reuptake inhibitors) are the most widely prescribed type of antidepressants.

Increasingly, people with moderate to severe depression are treated using a combination of antidepressants and CBT. Regular exercise has also been shown to be useful.

Cognitive behavioural therapy (CBT) helps to explore and change how you think about your life, and to free yourself from unhelpful patterns of behaviour. You set goals with your therapist and may carry out tasks between sessions.

Counselling is a form of talking therapy. A trained therapist listens to you and helps you find ways to deal with emotional issues.

Citalopram (brand name Cipramil) is an SSRI often used to treat depression and sometimes for panic attacks.

Depression makes you feel sad, hopeless and lose interest in activities you used to enjoy. Symptoms can persist for weeks or months and are bad enough to interfere with your work, social life and family life.

Diazepam (brand name Valium) is a medicine of the benzodiazepine family that can be very effective in treating the symptoms of anxiety, although it can't be used for long periods as it can become addictive.

Escitalopram (brand name Cipralex) is an SSRI often used to treat depression and sometimes for anxiety, obsessive compulsive disorder (OCD) or panic attacks.

Fluoxetine (brand name Prozac) is an SSRI often used to treat depression, and sometimes obsessive compulsive disorder and bulimia.

Mental health problems affect the way we think, feel and behave. 'Neurotic' covers those symptoms regarded as severe forms of 'normal' emotional experiences, such as depression, anxiety or panic. Less common are 'psychotic' symptoms, which interfere with a person's perception of reality, and may include hallucinations such as seeing, hearing, smelling or feeling things that no one else can. Mental health problems are usually defined and classified to enable professionals to refer people for appropriate care and treatment.

Oxazepam (originally branded as Serax) is a medicine of the benzodiazepine family. Oxazepam may be used for the short-term (maximum of two to four weeks) treatment of anxiety.

Quetiapine (brand names include Seroquel) is a second-generation (newer) antipsychotic drug that helps with conditions such as schizophrenia, mania and bipolar disorder.

A **psychiatrist** is a medical doctor and, unlike most practitioners, can prescribe medication when treating mental illness.

A **psychoanalyst** is the only practitioner that works with the unconscious – motivations and defence mechanisms that are out of our awareness, and therefore cause us to repeat harmful patterns.

A **psychologist** has a doctoral degree in psychology, which is the study of the mind and behaviours. Licensed psychologists are qualified to do counselling and psychotherapy, perform psychological testing, and provide treatment for mental disorders.

Psychotherapist is an umbrella term for any professional who is trained to treat people for their mental-health problems.

Sertraline (brand name Lustral) is an SSRI often used to treat depression, and sometimes panic attacks, obsessive compulsive disorder and post-traumatic stress disorder (PTSD).

Venlafaxine (brand names include Efexor XL) is often used to treat depression, and sometimes anxiety and panic attacks.

Sectioning in the UK means that you are kept in hospital under the Mental Health Act 1983. You can be sectioned if your own health or safety is at risk, or to protect other people.

SSRI stands for a selective serotonin reuptake inhibitor, a widely used type of antidepressant. SSRIs are usually the first choice medication for depression, because they generally have fewer side effects than most other types of antidepressant.

(Talking) therapy is a psychological treatment for mental and emotional problems like stress, anxiety and depression. There are different types, like CBT, and all involve working with a trained therapist. This may be one-to-one, in a group, over the phone, online, with your family, or with your partner. Usually there is little difference between counselling and talking (as opposed to drug) therapy.

Recommended Reading

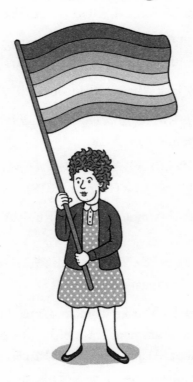

Mind Your Head by Juno Dawson (Hot Key Books, 2016)

Mad Girl: A Happy Life with a Mixed-Up Mind by Bryony Gordon (Headline, 2016)

How to Survive the End of the World (When it's in Your Own Head): An Anxiety Survival Guide by Aaron Gillies (Two Roads, 2018)

Reasons to Stay Alive by Matt Haig (Canongate Books, 2015)

The Colour of Madness: Exploring BAME Mental Health in the UK by Samara Linton, ed. (Skiddaw Books, 2018)

Making Winter: A Creative Guide for Surviving the Winter Months by Emma Mitchell (LOM Art, 2017)

Tin Can Cook by Jack Monroe (Bluebird, 2019)

Eat Up: Food, Appetite and Eating What You Want by Ruby Tandoh (Serpent's Tail, 2018)

Remember This When You're Sad: A Book for Mad, Sad and Glad Days by Maggy van Eijk (Lagom, 2018)

Sane New World: Taming the Mind by Ruby Wax (Hodder, 2014)

Insanely Gifted: Turn Your Demons into Creative Rocket Fuel by Jamie Catto (Canongate Books, 2017)

In addition, work by Mariko Tamaki, Craig Thompson, Neil Gaiman, Karrie Fransman, Dash Shaw, Adrian Tomine, Bryan and Mary Talbot, Alan Moore, Will Eisner, Art Spiegelman, and graphic reimaginings of classics like the Sherlock Holmes graphic novel series by Ian Edginton and I N J Culbard and everything that Marian Keyes has ever written.

Sources

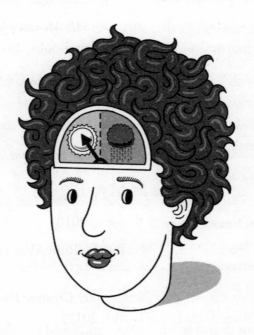

Preface

James Davies, *Cracked: Why Psychiatry is Doing More Harm than Good* (Icon Books, 2014)

Laura Donnelly and Patrick Scott, 'Pill nation: half of us take at least one prescription drug daily,' 2017, www.telegraph. co.uk/news/2017/12/13/pill-nation-half-us-take-least-one-prescription-drug-daily/

World Health Organization, 'Mental Health,' www.who.int/ mental_health/management/depression/en/

Mind, 'Mental health facts and statistics,' www.mind.org.uk/ information-support/types-of-mental-health-problems/ statistics-and-facts-about-mental-health/how-common-are-mental-health-problems/

Chapter 3: My shit job

My mental health story

Money Saving Expert, 'Mental health and debt,' www.moneysavingexpert.com/credit-cards/mental-health-guide/

Mental illness and work – your rights and entitlements

The Institute of Employment Rights, 'Unions and employers call for mental health to be given same weight as physical health,' 2018, www.ier.org.uk/news/unions-and-employers-call-mental-health-be-given-same-weight-physical-health/

Gwyn Topham, 'Make mental health as important as first aid, say business leaders,' 2018, www.theguardian.com/society/2018/nov/18/make-mental-health-important-first-aid-business-leaders-manifesto/

UK government, 'Taking sick leave,' www.gov.uk/taking-sick-leave/

Mind, 'Work is biggest cause of stress in people's lives,' 2013, www.mind.org.uk/news-campaigns/news/work-is-biggest-cause-of-stress-in-peoples-lives/

UK government, 'Reasonable adjustments for workers with disabilities or health conditions,' www.gov.uk/reasonable-adjustments-for-disabled-workers/

Rethink mental illness, 'Reasonable adjustments at work,' www.rethink.org/living-with-mental-illness/reasonable-adjustments-at-work/

UK government, 'Get help at work if you're disabled or have a health condition (Access to Work),' www.gov.uk/access-to-work/what-youll-get/

Chapter 4: My shit meds

NHS, 'Big new study confirms that antidepressants work better than placebo,' 2018, www.nhs.uk/news/medication/big-new-study-confirms-antidepressants-work-better-placebo/

Chapter 5: My shit therapist

TED, 'The power of vulnerability,' www.ted.com/talks/brene_
brown_on_vulnerability/

My actually-pretty-good therapist
UKCP, 'Common types of psychotherapy,' www.psychotherapy.
org.uk/about-psychotherapy/types/

How to choose your therapist
UK Council for Psychotherapy, www.psychotherapy.org.uk

British Association for Counselling and Psychotherapy,
www.bacp.co.uk

NHS Moodzone, 'Can I get free therapy or counselling?'
www.nhs.uk/conditions/stress-anxiety-depression/free-
therapy-or-counselling/

SANE, 'Textcare,' www.sane.org.uk/what_we_do/support/
textcare/

Mind, 'Apps for wellbeing and mental health,'
www.mindcharity.co.uk/advice-information/how-to-look-
after-your-mental-health/apps-for-wellbeing-and-mental-
health/

Chapter 6: My shit love life

Online dating
eHarmony, 'Over 50% of couples will meet online by 2031,'
www.eharmony.co.uk/dating-advice/online-dating-
unplugged/over-50-of-couples-will-meet-online-by-2031/

Hooked: How to Build Habit-Forming Products by Nir Eyal
(Portfolio Penguin, 2014)

Ryan O'Hare, 'Why the bright lights of a casino make
you bet more,' 2016, www.dailymail.co.uk/sciencetech/
article-3409991/Why-bright-lights-casino-make-bet-
Flashing-signs-disorientate-gamblers-causing-higher-risks.
html/

Henry Blodget, '90% of 18–29 year olds sleep with their
smartphones,' 2012, www.businessinsider.com/90-of-18-29-
year-olds-sleep-with-their-smartphones-2012-11/

University of North Texas, 'Men have highest risk for low self-
esteem while using Tinder, UNT study finds,' 2016, https://
news.unt.edu/news-releases/men-have-highest-risk-low-
self-esteem-while-using-tinder-unt-study-finds/

Sam Levin, 'Facebook told advertisers it can identify teens
feeling "insecure" and "worthless",' 2017, www.theguardian.
com/technology/2017/may/01/facebook-advertising-data-
insecure-teens/

American Psychological Association, 'Tinder: swiping self-
esteem?', 2016, www.apa.org/news/press/releases/2016/08/
tinder-self-esteem.aspx/

E Timmermans, E de Caluwé, C Alexopoulos, 'Why are you
cheating on Tinder? Exploring users' motives and (dark)
personality traits', Computers in Human Behaviour, Vol
89, pp 129–39, December 2018, www.sciencedirect.com/
science/article/pii/S0747563218303625

B A Liu yi Lin et al, 'Association between social media use and depression among US young adults', Depression & Anxiety, 2016, 33(4): 323–331, www.ncbi.nlm.nih.gov/pmc/articles/PMC4853817/

Single, and please don't make me mingle
Edith Hancock, 'These are the secrets to long life, according to 5 of the oldest people in the world,' 2016, www.independent.co.uk/life-style/these-are-the-secrets-to-long-life-according-to-5-of-the-oldest-people-in-the-world-a7465766.html/

Chapter 7: My shit body

Body issues
NHS, 'Overview: obesity,' www.nhs.uk/conditions/obesity/

My first 10k
Nicola Kemp, 'Case study: How 'This girl can' got 1.6 million women exercising,' 2016, www.campaignlive.co.uk/article/case-study-this-girl-can-16-million-women-exercising/1394836/

Brittaney Kiefer, 'Sport England's "This girl can" returns to encourage unconventional forms of exercise,' 2018, www.campaignlive.co.uk/article/sport-englands-this-girl-can-returns-encourage-unconventional-forms-exercise/1497206/

Chapter 8: My shit habits

Centre for Mental Health, 'Mental health problems at work cost UK economy £34.9bn last year, says Centre for Mental Health,' www.centreformentalhealth.org.uk/news/mental-health-problems-work-cost-uk-economy-ps349bn-last-year-says-centre-mental-health/

Chapter 9: My shit home

Zoopla property news team, 'The average Brit "will move house eight times",' 2012, www.zoopla.co.uk/discover/property-news/the-average-brit-will-move-house-8-times-801377088/

Rhiannon Lucy Cosslett, '"I have sleepless nights": the looming mental health crisis facing generation rent,' 2018, www.theguardian.com/society/2018/may/09/mental-health-crisis-generation-rent-millennials-own-home-wellbeing/

Chapter 10: My brilliant shit brain

The big, sexy ending

The Seven Basic Plots: Why we tell stories by Christopher Booker (Continuum, 2004)

Glossary

www.nhs.uk/medicines/
www.nhs.uk/medicines/

www.mind.org.uk/information-support/drugs-and-treatments/

www.mentalhealth.org.uk/your-mental-health/about-mental-health/what-are-mental-health-problems/

www.psychologytoday.com/ca/blog/couch-meets-world/201107/psychiatrist-psychotherapist-whos-who-in-mental-health/

www.webmd.com/mental-health/guide-to-psychiatry-and-counseling

www.mind.org.uk/information-support/legal-rights/sectioning/

Acknowledgements

First and foremost, I thank each contributor who trusted me with their mental health stories and allowed me to share them in this book. I also thank every one of my followers, who've been cheering me on since I worked in a cafe and wrote a blog post that flew around the world. I can't tell you what your support means to me. I hope I've done you proud. Thank you to my family and friends for your boundless and unreserved love.

To my agents, Sophie and Emma, and all at Bonnier Books UK, especially Natalie, Beth, Caroline, and Kate, and my formidably brilliant editor Sadie Mayne.

Diolch o galon. xx